JUICING FOR CANCER

RECIPES BOOK FOR SENIORS

75+ Delicious and Healthy Juicing Recipes to Boost Your Immune System, Fight Inflammation, and Improve Your Health

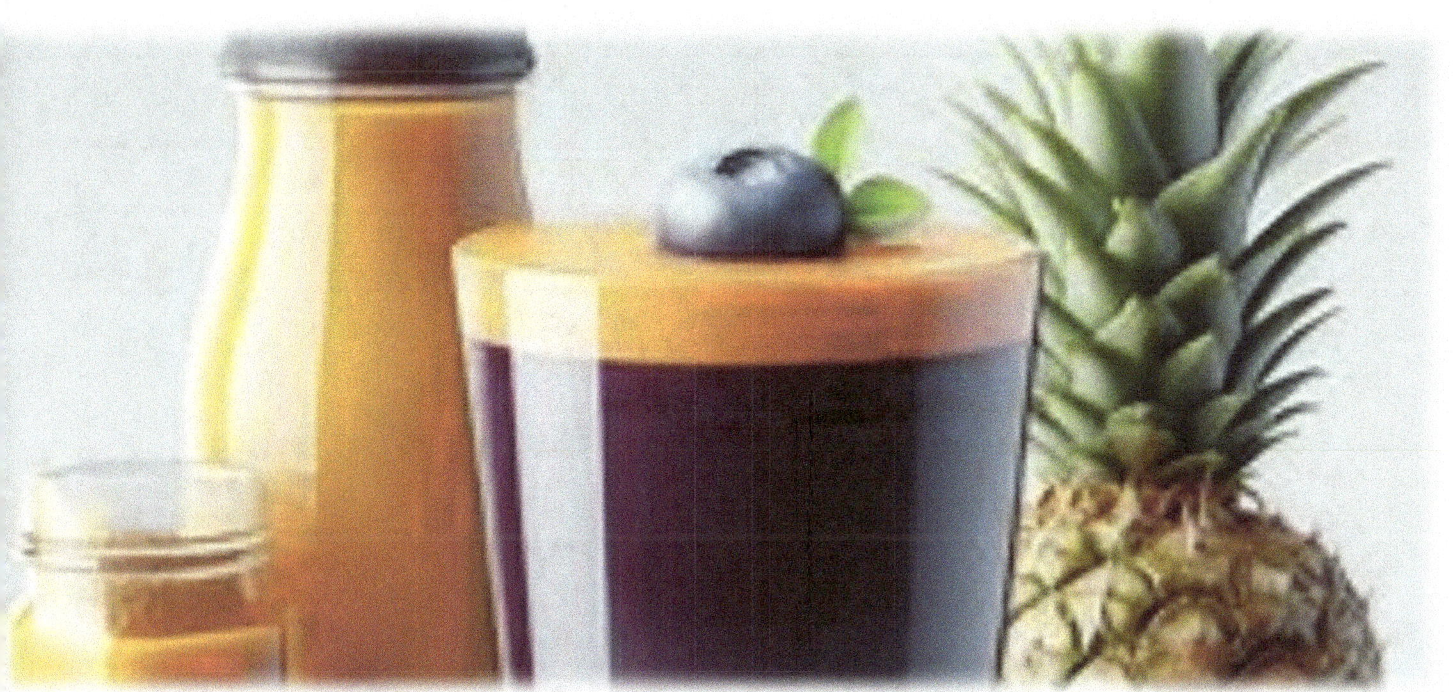

By Sharon D. Newsome

Copyright© 2024 by Sharon D. Newsome

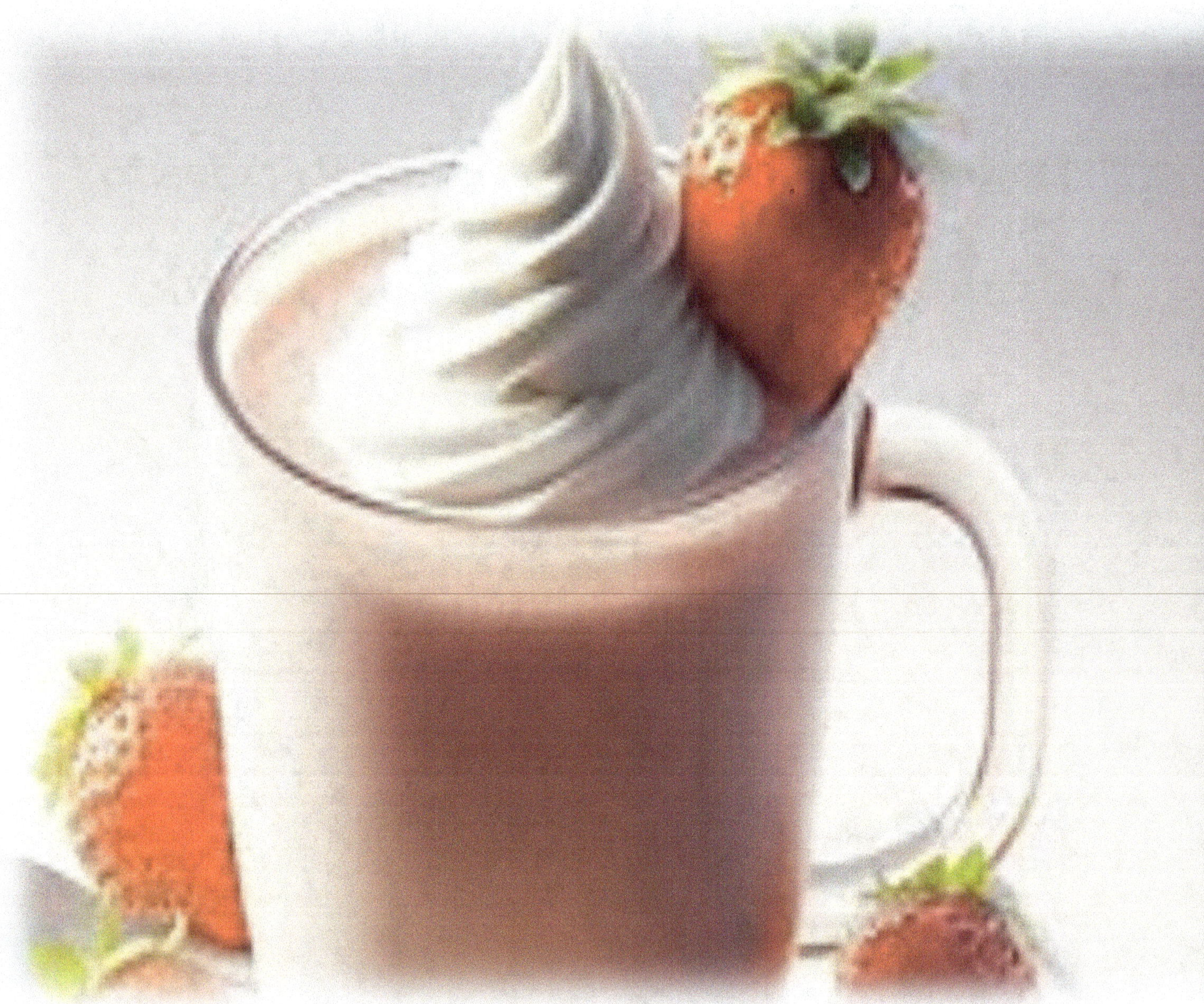

   Juicing for Cancer Recipes for Seniors

TABLE OF CONTENTS

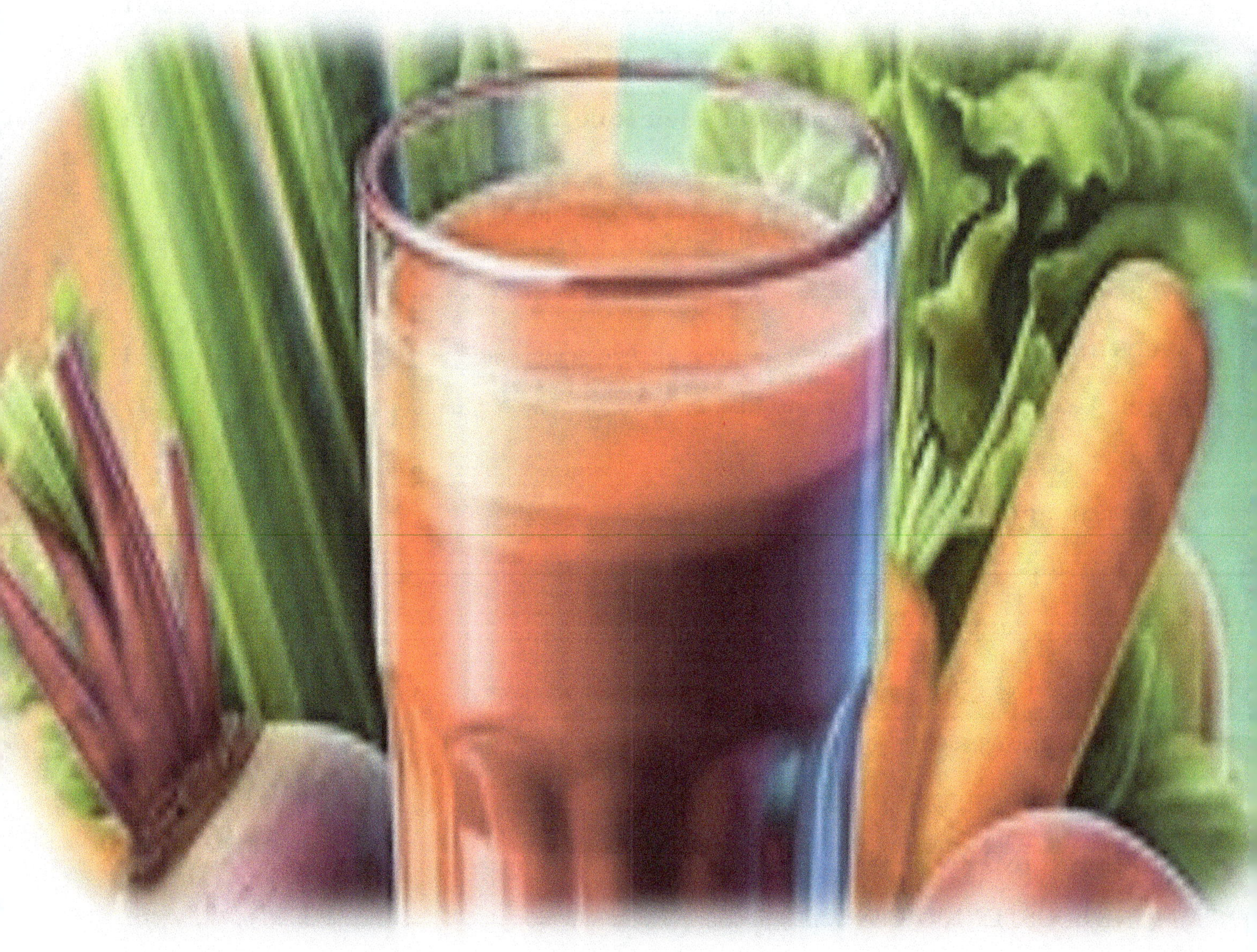

INTRODUCTION

Emilia, a 65-year-old woman who had been diagnosed with breast cancer two years ago. She had gone through surgery, chemotherapy, and radiation therapy, but the cancer had spread to her bones and lungs. Emilia was feeling weak, tired, and depressed and had lost her appetite and weight. Her doctor had told her that there was not much more they could do for her and also told her to try as much as she could to enjoy every bit of the remaining time of her life.

One day, her daughter came to visit her with a book about juicing for cancer. Her daughter explained that she had found the book online and that it might help her mother feel better. She said that the book contained recipes of juices that are specially designed for seniors who were diagnosed with cancer or undergoing cancer treatment. The juices were supposed to provide nutrients, antioxidants, enzymes, and water that could boost the immune system, increase energy levels, improve digestion, detoxify the body, and reduce inflammation and pain.

Emilia was full of doubt at first, but on a second thought, he made up her mind to try it out. She asked her daughter to buy a juicer and some fruits and vegetables. She started with the book's first recipe. She was surprised by how refreshing and energizing it tasted. She felt a warm sensation in her throat and stomach and a slight tingling in her fingers and toes. She drank the juice every morning for a week and noticed that she had more appetite and less nausea.

She then moved on to the second recipe. She loved the sweet and tart flavor of the berries and the creamy texture of the flaxseed. She felt more alert and focused and less depressed. She drank the juice every afternoon for a week and noticed that she had more stamina and less fatigue.

She followed the book's recipes, trying different combinations of fruits and vegetables daily. She experimented with lemons, grapefruits, apples, kale, cabbage, celery, cucumbers, pineapples, pears, prunes, beets, broccoli, garlic, mint, cilantro, green tea, cayenne pepper, and more. She enjoyed the juices' variety of colors, flavors, and aromas. Emilia felt more hydrated, fresher, and lighter.

After a month of juicing, she returned to her doctor for a check-up. She was amazed by the results. Her blood tests showed that her white blood cell count, hemoglobin level, and liver function had improved. Her tumor markers had decreased.

Her bone scan showed that the density of her bone had increased. Her chest X-ray showed that her lung nodules had shrunk. Her doctor was astonished by her progress. He said he had never seen such a remarkable improvement in such a short time. He asked her what she had been doing differently. She told him about the book and the juices.

He congratulated her on her success and encouraged her to keep juicing. He said he would recommend the book to his other patients in similar situations. He noted that juicing might not be a cure, but it could certainly help improve the quality of life.

Emilia thanked him for his support and hugged her daughter, who was waiting outside. She felt a surge of gratitude, hope, and joy. From then on, Emilia realized that juicing had helped her physically, mentally, and emotionally. She felt more connected to herself, to nature, and to life.

She decided to write a testimonial for the book and share her story with others who might benefit from it. She wanted to inspire them to try juicing and experience its healing power.

Juicing is a simple and effective way to nourish your body and mind with nature's gifts. It is a way to celebrate life and enjoy its beauty and bounty, way to show yourself some love and care. It is also a way to juice up your health and happiness.

Juicing is not a miracle cure for cancer or any other disease. It is not to be used to replace medical advice or treatment. There is a variety of solutions for some seniors.

Speaking with your doctor or nutritionist before starting any juicing plan is vital, especially if you have any medical concerns or use drugs that may interfere with specific nutrients or components. Remember to regularly check your blood sugar levels, blood pressure, and weight. It would help to balance your juicing intake with other healthy foods and beverages.

CHAPTER ONE

UNDERSTANDING CANCER AND NUTRITION

Juicing for cancer is an excellent method for obtaining a concentrated dosage of nutrients from fruits and vegetables. Juicing can help to boost the immune system, reduce inflammation, and fight off cancer cells.

Fruits and veggies are rich in vitamins, fiber, antioxidants, minerals, and other phytonutrients proven to have cancer-fighting properties. For example, berries are high in anthocyanins, which have antioxidant and anti-inflammatory effects. Glucosinolates are found in cruciferous plants such as broccoli and cauliflower and convert into compounds that help fight cancer cells. Fresh citrus fruits provide a lot of vitamin C, which can help improve immunity.

When you juice fruits and veggies, you eliminate the insoluble fiber, making the nutrients more easily absorbed by the body. This can be especially beneficial for people with cancer, who may have digestive problems that make it difficult to absorb nutrients from food.

Cancer is a formidable adversary, a term that often fills our thoughts with concern and uncertainty. To understand how nutrition can play a crucial role in the fight against cancer, we must first grasp the nature of this relentless disease.

What is Cancer?

Cancer, in its essence, is a battle within our bodies. It results from cells that have gone astray, losing their natural control mechanisms. Cells divide and grow orderly in a healthy body, then die at a set time. However, when the DNA, the genetic code within a cell, becomes damaged or altered, it can lead to uncontrolled cell growth.

This uncontrolled cell growth can give rise to a mass of tissue known as a tumor. Tumors can interfere with the body's natural processes and take up space and nutrients needed for normal cell function. Not all tumors are cancerous. Benign tumors don't spread, while malignant tumors invade nearby tissues and even distant organs in a process called metastasis.

It's essential to recognize that cancer is not a single, uniform disease; it encompasses a wide range of conditions. There are over 100 types of cancer, each with unique characteristics and behaviors. For instance, breast cancer differs significantly from lung cancer, and leukemia is distinct from melanoma. However, they all share a common feature: the uncontrolled growth of abnormal cells.

The Connection between Diet and Cancer

The link between our diet and cancer has been the subject of extensive research, and the findings are compelling. While no diet can guarantee immunity from cancer, the food we choose to consume has a profound impact on our physical well-being. It can significantly influence our susceptibility to cancer.

Understanding the nature of cancer is the first step in our journey towards using nutrition as a powerful tool to complement cancer treatment and support the well-being of patients. As we move forward, we'll explore the intricate connection between diet and cancer, and we'll go deeper into the specific nutritional needs of those battling this formidable adversary.

Nutritional Needs for Cancer Patients

Numerous studies have shown that certain dietary habits can either increase or decrease the likelihood of developing cancer. Diets high in processed foods, sugary beverages, processed and red meats, and low in fruits, vegetables, and whole grains are associated with an elevated risk of cancer. On the contrary, eating a diet rich in fruits, vegetables, nutritious grains, and lean meats is an effective method to protect yourself against cancer.

Cancer and its treatments can exert a toll on the body, affecting nutritional requirements and creating unique challenges. Understanding these needs is crucial for individuals battling cancer.

1. Caloric and Protein Requirements

Cancer patients often have increased calorie and protein needs. The body's energy expenditure can rise due to the disease's demands and treatments' effects. Moreover, protein is essential for repairing and maintaining body tissues, especially during illness. Patients need to ensure they are getting adequate calories and protein to support their overall health and recovery.

2. Micronutrients and Antioxidants

Many cancer patients may experience deficiencies in essential vitamins and minerals due to poor appetite, side effects of treatment, or impaired nutrient absorption. Micronutrients like vitamin D, B12, and iron are of particular concern. Antioxidant compounds like vitamins C and E are also essential to protect cells from harm caused by oxidative stress.

3. Hydration

Staying well-hydrated is essential for cancer patients, especially if they experience side effects like diarrhea, vomiting, or increased perspiration. Dehydration can worsen these symptoms and lead to more significant health issues. Drinking adequate fluids is crucial for maintaining overall well-being during cancer treatment.

4. Managing Side Effects

Cancer treatments can cause various side effects, including changes in taste, nausea, and difficulty swallowing. Understanding how to manage these side effects through proper nutrition is essential. For instance, choosing bland or cold foods may help reduce nausea, and specific strategies can help maintain adequate nutrition even when eating becomes challenging.

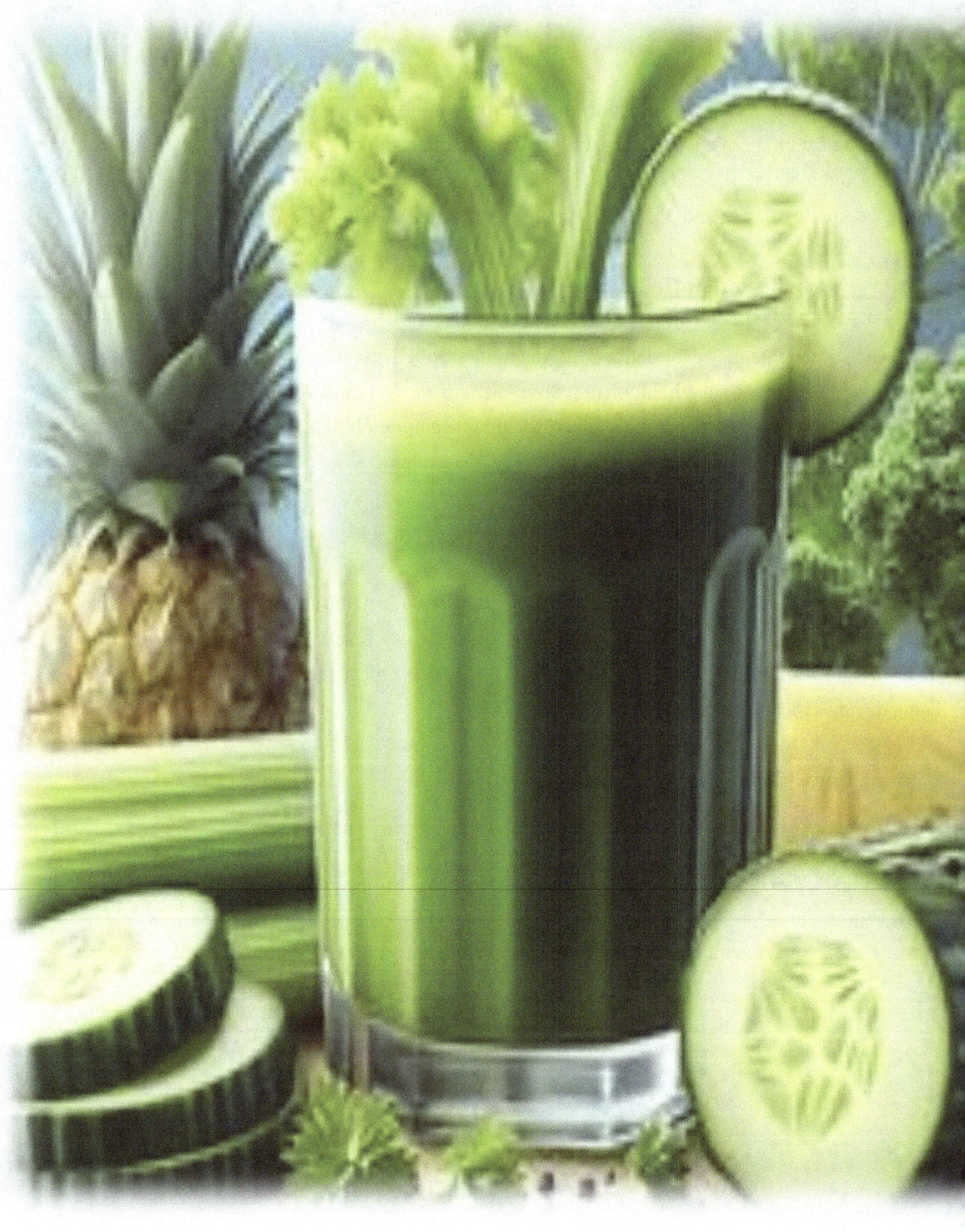

 Juicing for Cancer Recipes for Seniors

CHAPTER TWO

BENEFITS OF JUICING FOR CANCER

Every advantage matters when it comes to the difficult path of cancer treatment. Juicing offers unique benefits that can support cancer patients during their treatment and recovery. The essence of juicing lies in creating concentrated, nutrient-packed concoctions from fresh fruits, vegetables, and herbs. These vibrant elixirs offer several advantages:

1. Enhances Nutrient Absorption

Cancer treatments can sometimes affect the digestive system, making it challenging for the body to absorb nutrients effectively. Juices are a great way to provide easily digestible, concentrated nutrition, ensuring the body gets the vital vitamins, minerals, and antioxidants it needs.

2. It Helps with Hydration and Nourishment

Many cancer treatments can lead to side effects such as nausea loss of appetite, and can cause dehydration and malnutrition. Maintaining proper hydration is crucial. Juices, often brimming with water content, can help in staying hydrated.

3. Supports the Immune System

Cancer treatment often weakens the immune system. Juices brimming with antioxidants and immune-boosting nutrients can fortify the body's defenses, helping it fight infections and recover more effectively.

4. Reduces Inflammation and Oxidative Stress

Inflammation and oxidative stress are two processes in the body that can contribute to cancer development. An unhealthy diet, especially one high in processed and fatty foods, can promote chronic inflammation and lead to an increased risk of cancer. Foods rich in antioxidants, like veggies and colorful fruits, can help fight toxic stress and inflammation, lowering the risk.

5. Maintain a Healthy Weight

Obesity is very risky for various types of cancer, including breast, colon, and prostate cancer. Therefore, a diet that promotes weight management is essential for cancer prevention. A healthy, well-balanced food and daily exercise may be very good for our health. This can help you keep a good weight and lower your cancer risk. We must prioritize our health and incorporate these changes into our daily lives.

The Use of Nutrient-Rich Ingredients for Juicing

One of the cornerstones of juicing for cancer patients is using nutrient-dense ingredients. These ingredients provide a concentrated source of essential vitamins and minerals to aid recovery and well-being.

1. Fruits: Fresh fruits like oranges, berries, and kiwi contain essential vitamins and antioxidants. Citrus fruits, for instance, provide Vitamin C, which boosts the immune system and assists in the formation of collagen.

2. Vegetables: Leafy greens like spinach and kale contain vitamins like A, C, and K and minerals like iron and calcium. These nutrients are essential for strong bones, good skin, and a robust immune system.

3. Herbs: Herbs like basil, cilantro, and parsley are flavorful additions to your juices and offer unique phytochemicals and antioxidants that can support your body's natural defense mechanisms.

Antioxidants, Phytochemicals, and Their Role

Antioxidants and phytochemicals are the unsung heroes in the world of nutrition, and they play a vital role in cancer prevention and treatment.

Antioxidants

Antioxidants safeguard cells against the oxidative stress caused by free radicals.

Free radicals can harm cells, leading to various health problems, including cancer. Juices loaded with antioxidants from ingredients like blueberries, cherries, and green tea can assist in neutralizing these harmful compounds.

Phytochemicals

Phytochemicals are naturally occurring substances found in plants. Many of them were studied for their potential to prevent and treat cancer. For example, resveratrol in grapes, lycopene in tomatoes, and curcumin in turmeric are well-known phytochemicals with promising anticancer properties.

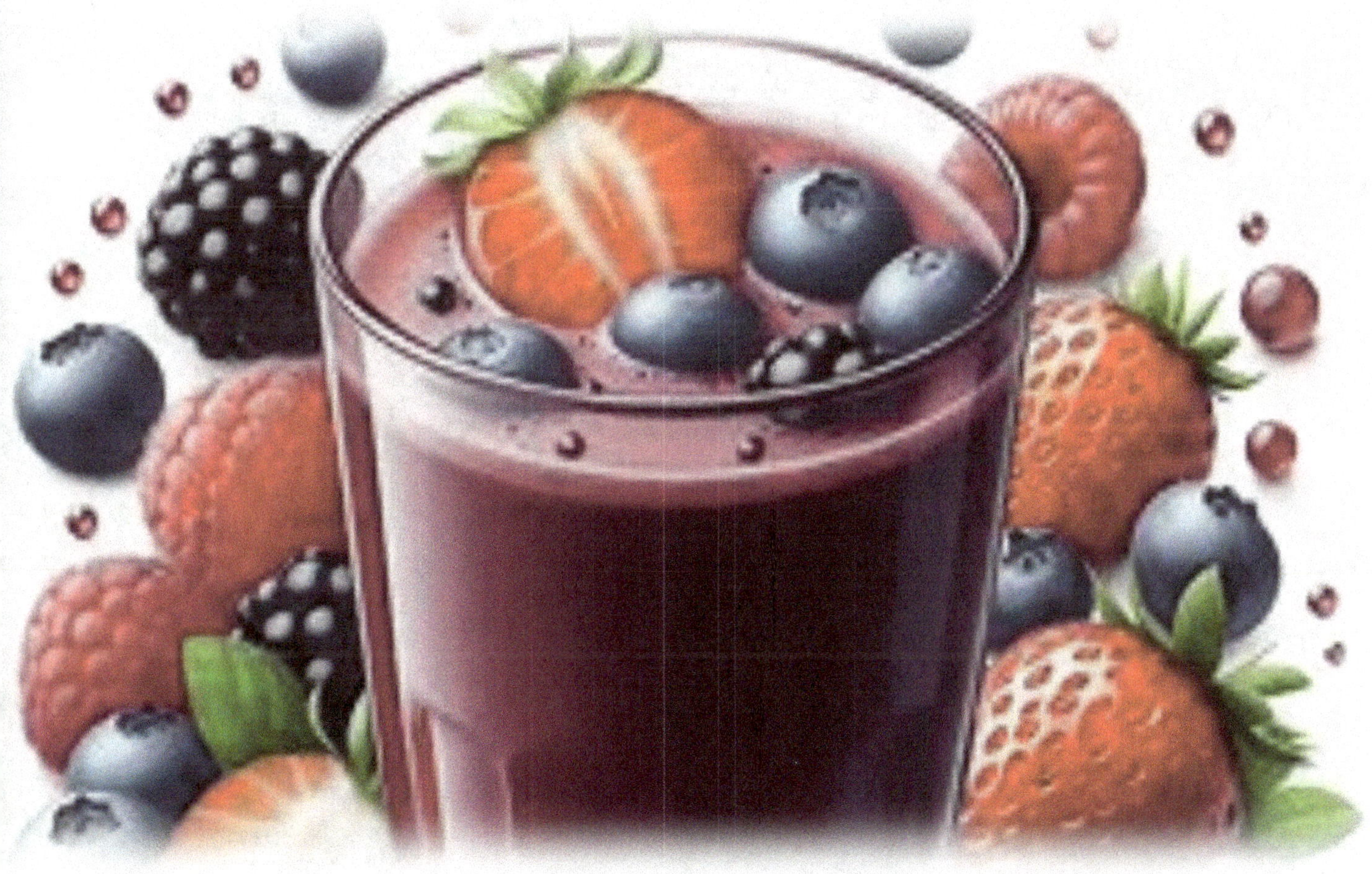

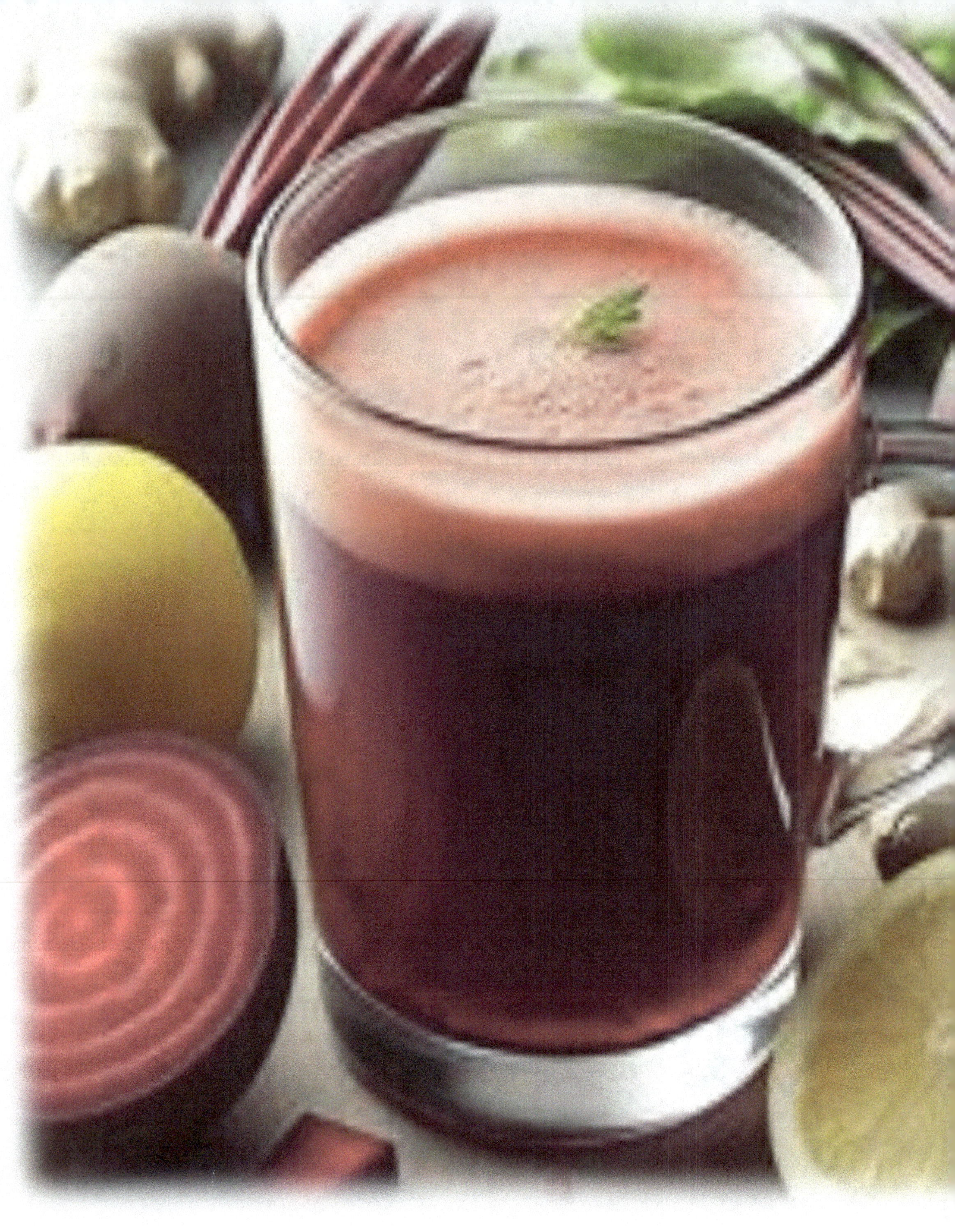

 Juicing for Cancer Recipes for Seniors

<h1 style="text-align:center">CHAPTER THREE</h1>

A 28-Day Meal Plan for Cancer Patients

Week 1

Breakfast

Day 1: Oatmeal with berries and nuts, plus The Berry Bliss juice

Day 2: Yogurt with fruit and granola, plus The Green Goddess juice

Day 3: Scrambled eggs with vegetables, plus The Turmeric Tonic juice

Day 4: Smoothie made with berries, yoghurt, and chia seeds, plus The Watermelon Warrior juice

Day 5: Whole-wheat toast with avocado and eggs, plus The Golden Glow juice

Day 6: Pancakes with fruit and yoghurt, plus The Tropical Oasis juice

Day 7: Omelet with vegetables and cheese, plus The Beet Blast juice

Lunch

Day 1: Grilled chicken or fish salad, plus The Berry Bliss juice

Day 2: Soup and sandwich, plus The Green Goddess juice

Day 3: Leftovers from dinner, plus The Turmeric Tonic juice

Day 4: Tuna salad sandwich on whole-wheat bread, plus The Watermelon Warrior juice

Day 5: Salad with quinoa and chickpeas, plus The Golden Glow juice

Day 6: Leftovers from dinner, plus The Tropical Oasis juice

Day 7: Lentil soup, plus The Beet Blast juice

Dinner

Day 1: Grilled salmon with roasted vegetables, plus The Golden Glow juice

Day 2: Chicken stir-fry with brown rice, plus The Green Goddess juice

Day 3: Lentil soup, plus The Turmeric Tonic juice

Day 4: Spaghetti with Bolognese sauce, plus The Watermelon Warrior juice

Day 5: Chicken fajitas with brown rice and vegetables, plus The Tropical Oasis juice

Day 6: Roasted chicken with roasted vegetables, plus The Beet Blast juice

Day 7: Vegetarian chili, plus The Berry Bliss juice

Snacks

Fruits and vegetables

Nuts and seeds

Yogurt

Hard-boiled eggs

Whole-wheat crackers

Hard cheese

Juices from the recipes above

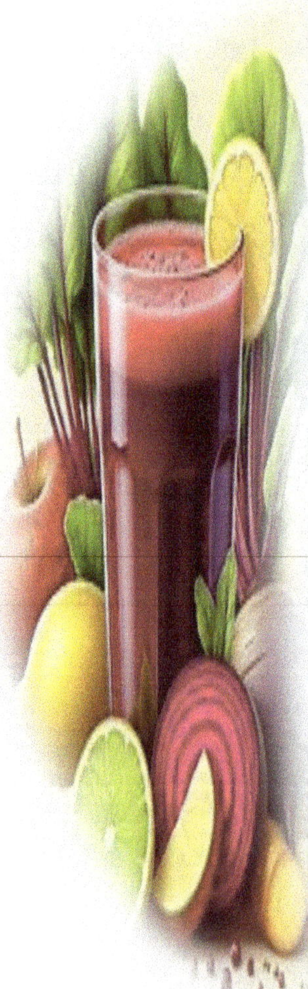

Week 2

Breakfast

Day 1: Smoothie made with berries, yogurt, and chia seeds, plus The Golden Glow juice

Day 2: Oatmeal with nuts and seeds, plus The Green Goddess juice

Day 3: Yogurt with fruit and granola, plus The Turmeric Tonic juice

Day 4: Scrambled eggs with vegetables, plus The Watermelon Warrior juice

Day 5: Toast with avocado and eggs, plus The Tropical Oasis juice

Day 6: Pancakes with fruit and yogurt, plus The Beet Blast juice

Day 7: Omelet with vegetables and cheese, plus The Berry Bliss juice

Lunch

Day 1: Grilled chicken or fish salad, plus The Turmeric Tonic juice

Day 2: Soup and sandwich, plus The Watermelon Warrior juice

Day 3: Leftovers from dinner, plus The Tropical Oasis juice

Day 4: Tuna salad sandwich on whole-wheat bread, plus The Beet Blast juice

Day 5: Salad with quinoa and chickpeas, plus The Berry Bliss juice

Day 6: Leftovers from dinner, plus The Golden Glow juice

Day 7: Lentil soup, plus The Green Goddess juice

Dinner

Day 1: Shrimp scampi with whole-wheat pasta, plus The Green Goddess juice

Day 2: Tofu stir-fry with brown rice, plus The Turmeric Tonic juice

Day 3: Chicken pot pie, plus The Watermelon Warrior juice

Day 4: Beef stew, plus The Tropical Oasis juice

Day 5: Fish tacos with brown rice and vegetables, plus The Beet Blast juice

Day 6: Turkey meatballs with spaghetti squash, plus The Berry Bliss juice

Day 7: Vegetarian lasagna, plus The Golden Glow juice

Snacks

Fruits and vegetables

Nuts and seeds

Yogurt

Hard-boiled eggs

Whole-wheat crackers

Hard cheese

Juices from the recipes above

Week 3

Breakfast

Day 1: Toast with avocado and eggs, plus The Green Goddess juice

Day 2: Oatmeal with nuts and seeds, plus The Turmeric Tonic juice

Day 3: Yogurt with fruit and granola, plus The Watermelon Warrior juice

Day 4: Scrambled eggs with vegetables, plus The Tropical Oasis juice

Day 5: Pancakes with fruit and yogurt, plus The Beet Blast juice

Day 6: Omelet with vegetables and cheese, plus The Berry Bliss juice

Day 7: Smoothie made with berries, yogurt, and chia seeds, plus The Golden Glow juice

Lunch

Day 1: Grilled chicken or fish salad, plus The Watermelon Warrior juice

Week 3

Lunch

Day 1: Grilled chicken or fish salad, plus The Watermelon Warrior juice

Day 2: Soup and sandwich, plus The Tropical Oasis juice

Day 3: Leftovers from dinner, plus The Beet Blast juice

Day 4: Tuna salad sandwich on whole-wheat bread, plus The Berry Bliss juice

Day 5: Salad with quinoa and chickpeas, plus The Golden Glow juice

Day 6: Leftovers from dinner, plus The Green Goddess juice

Day 7: Lentil soup, plus The Turmeric Tonic juice

Dinner

Day 1: Grilled steak with roasted vegetables, plus The Tropical Oasis juice

Day 2: Chicken curry with brown rice, plus The Beet Blast juice

Day 3: Lentil soup, plus The Berry Bliss juice

Day 4: Salmon with roasted vegetables, plus The Golden Glow juice

Day 5: Pork chops with mashed potatoes and green beans, plus The Green Goddess juice

Day 6: Vegetarian chili, plus The Turmeric Tonic juice

Day 7: Chicken fajitas with brown rice and vegetables, plus The Watermelon Warrior juice

Snacks

Fruits and vegetables

Nuts and seeds

Yogurt

Hard-boiled eggs

Whole-wheat crackers

Hard cheese

Juices from the recipes above

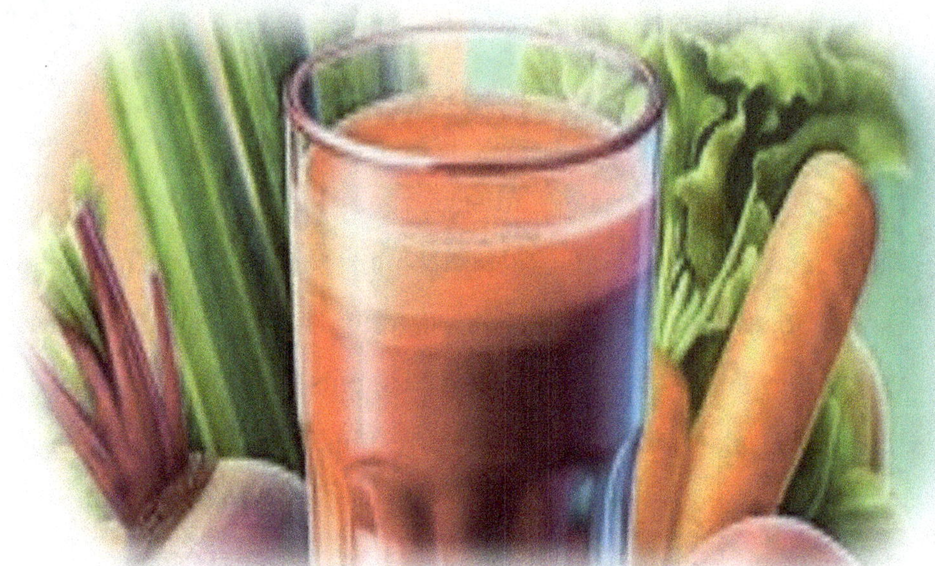

Week 4

Breakfast

Day 1: Pancakes with fruit and yogurt, plus The Beet Blast juice

Day 2: Oatmeal with nuts and seeds, plus The Berry Bliss juice

Day 3: Yogurt with fruit and granola, plus The Golden Glow juice

Day 4: Scrambled eggs with vegetables, plus The Green Goddess juice

Day 5: Toast with avocado and eggs, plus The Turmeric Tonic juice

Day 6: Omelet with vegetables and cheese, plus The Watermelon Warrior juice

Day 7: Smoothie made with berries, yogurt, and chia seeds, plus The Tropical Oasis juice

Lunch

Day 1: Grilled chicken or fish salad, plus The Berry Bliss juice

 Juicing for Cancer Recipes for Seniors

Day 2: Soup and sandwich, plus The Golden Glow juice

Day 3: Leftovers from dinner, plus The Green Goddess juice

Day 4: Tuna salad sandwich on whole-wheat bread, plus The Turmeric Tonic juice

Day 5: Salad with quinoa and chickpeas, plus The Watermelon Warrior juice

Day 6: Leftovers from dinner, plus The Tropical Oasis juice

Day 7: Lentil soup, plus The Beet Blast juice

Dinner

Day 1: Chicken parmesan with spaghetti squash, plus The Green Goddess juice

Day 2: Shrimp scampi with whole-wheat pasta, plus The Turmeric Tonic juice

Day 3: Vegetarian lasagna, plus The Watermelon Warrior juice

Day 4: Beef stew, plus The Tropical Oasis juice

Day 5: Turkey meatballs with spaghetti squash, plus The Beet Blast juice

Day 6: Fish tacos with brown rice and vegetables, plus The Berry Bliss juice

Day 7: Tofu stir-fry with brown rice, plus The Golden Glow juice

Snacks

Fruits and vegetables

Nuts and seeds

Yogurt

Hard-boiled eggs

Whole-wheat crackers

Hard cheese

Juices from the recipes above

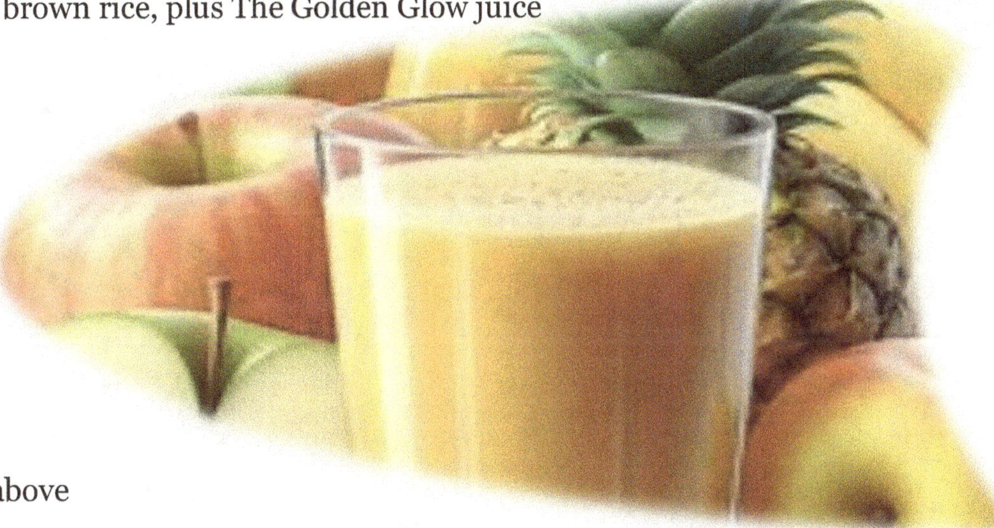

This meal plan is only a guideline; you can modify it to meet your nutritional needs and tastes. Before making any substantial dietary changes, consult your doctor or a trained nutritionist.

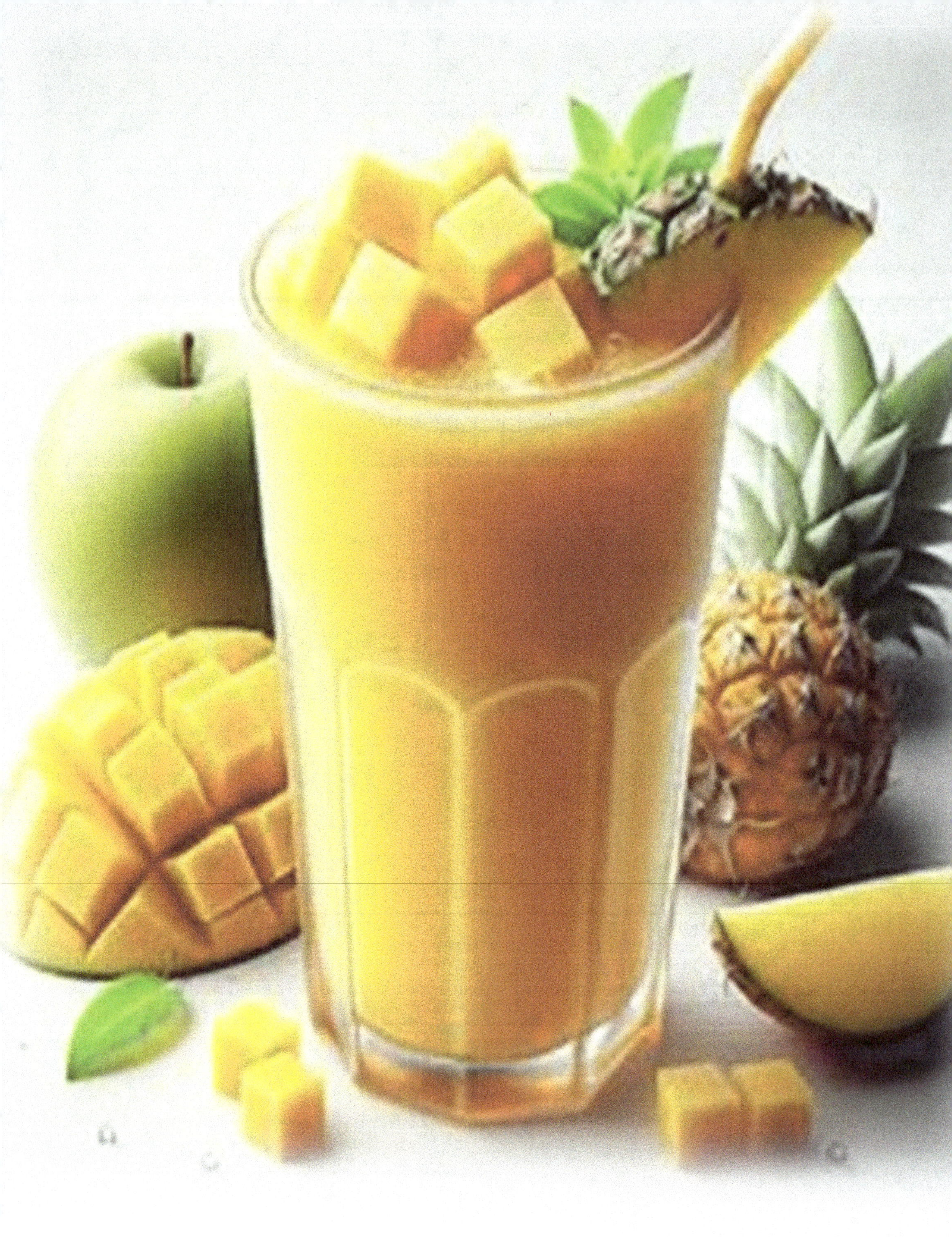

 Juicing for Cancer Recipes for Seniors

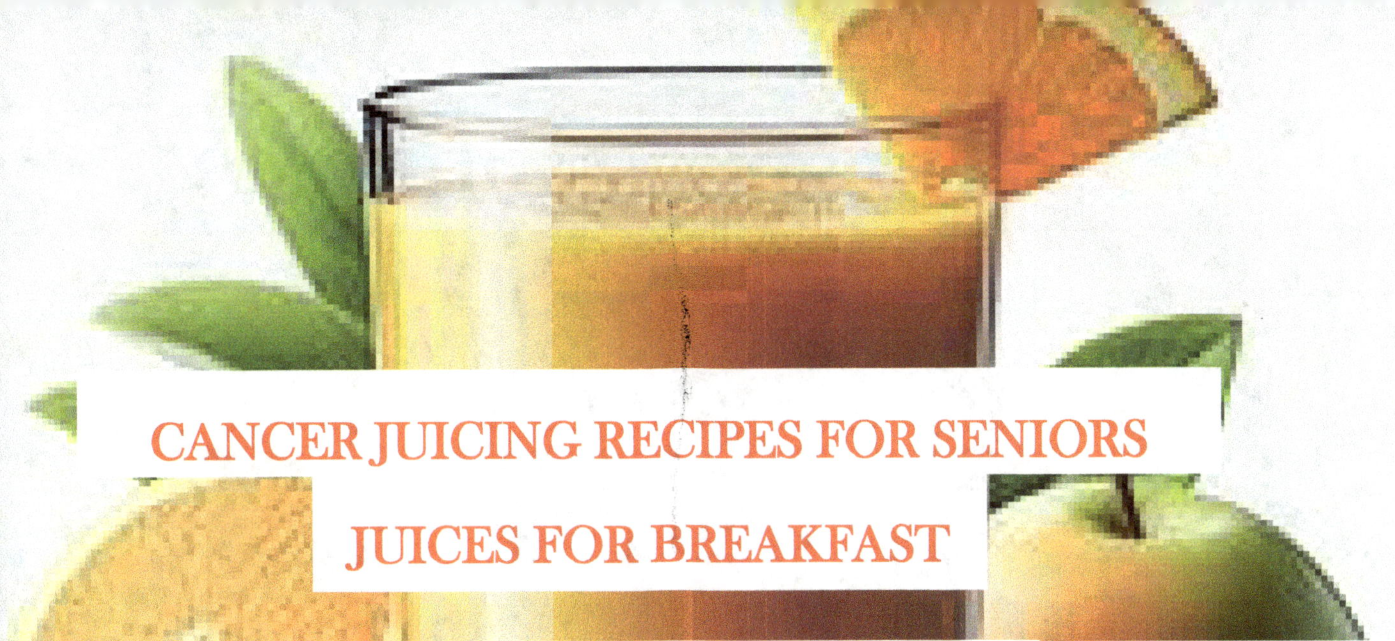

1.   The Antioxidant Rich

Introduction:

This juice contains essential vitamins and minerals for a healthy breakfast. Carrots, oranges, and mango provide vitamins A and C, while ginger and turmeric have anti-inflammatory and antioxidant properties.

Ingredients:

1 cup carrots

1 orange, peeled and segmented

1/2 cup mango, peeled and diced

1/2 inch peeled and chopped ginger root

1/4 inch turmeric root, peeled and chopped

Instructions:

Wash all of the ingredients well.

Cut the carrots and mango into small pieces.

Add all of the ingredients to a juicer and blend until smooth.

Serve immediately.

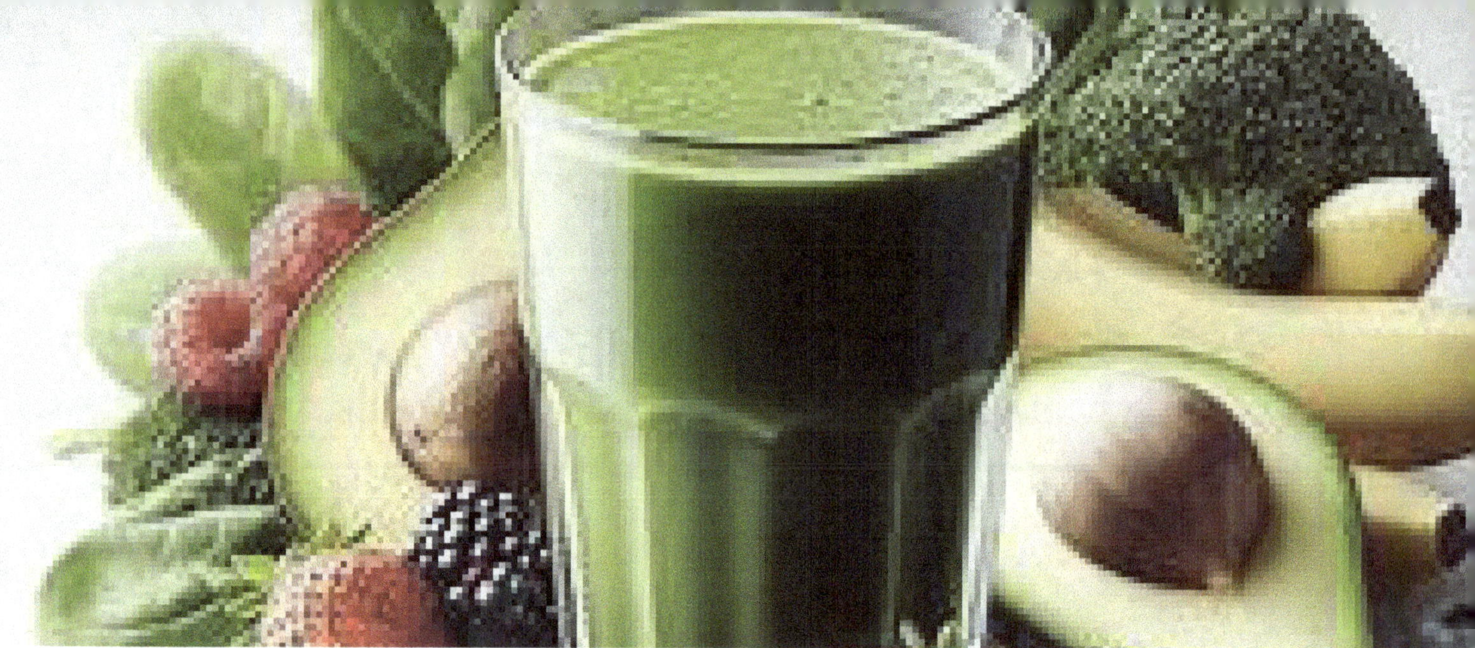

2. Green Smoothie juice

Introduction:

This smoothie is a great way to start your day with a boost of nutrients. The spinach, kale, and avocado are packed with vitamins, minerals, and healthy fats. The banana and berries add sweetness and creaminess.

Ingredients:

1 cup spinach

1 cup kale

1/2 avocado

1 banana

1/2 cup berries (any kind)

1 cup almond milk

Instructions:

Wash all of the ingredients well.

Cut the banana into small pieces.

Include all the ingredients in a blender and blend until smooth.

Serve immediately.

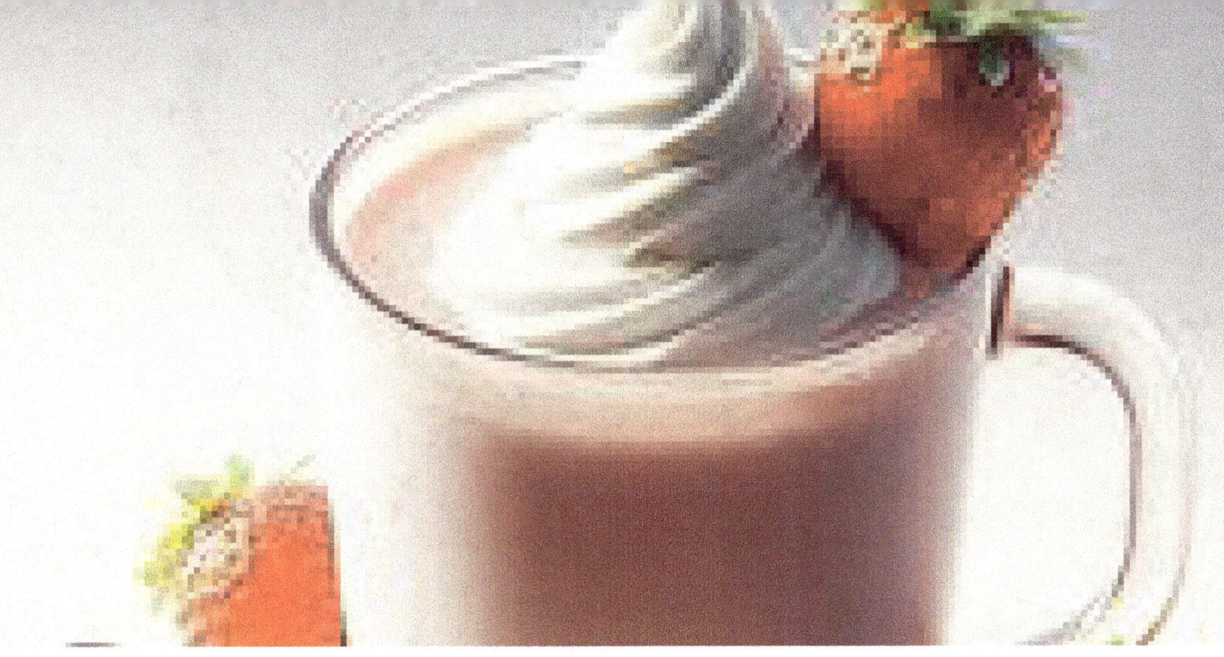

3. Berry Blast juice

Introduction:

This juice is packed with vitamins and antioxidants, making it an excellent choice for breakfast. The berries provide vitamins A, C, and K, while the yogurt adds protein and probiotics.

Ingredients:

1 cup berries (any kind)

1 cup yogurt (plain or Greek)

1/2 cup milk (any type)

Instructions:

Wash all of the ingredients well.

Include all the ingredients in a blender and blend until smooth.

Serve immediately.

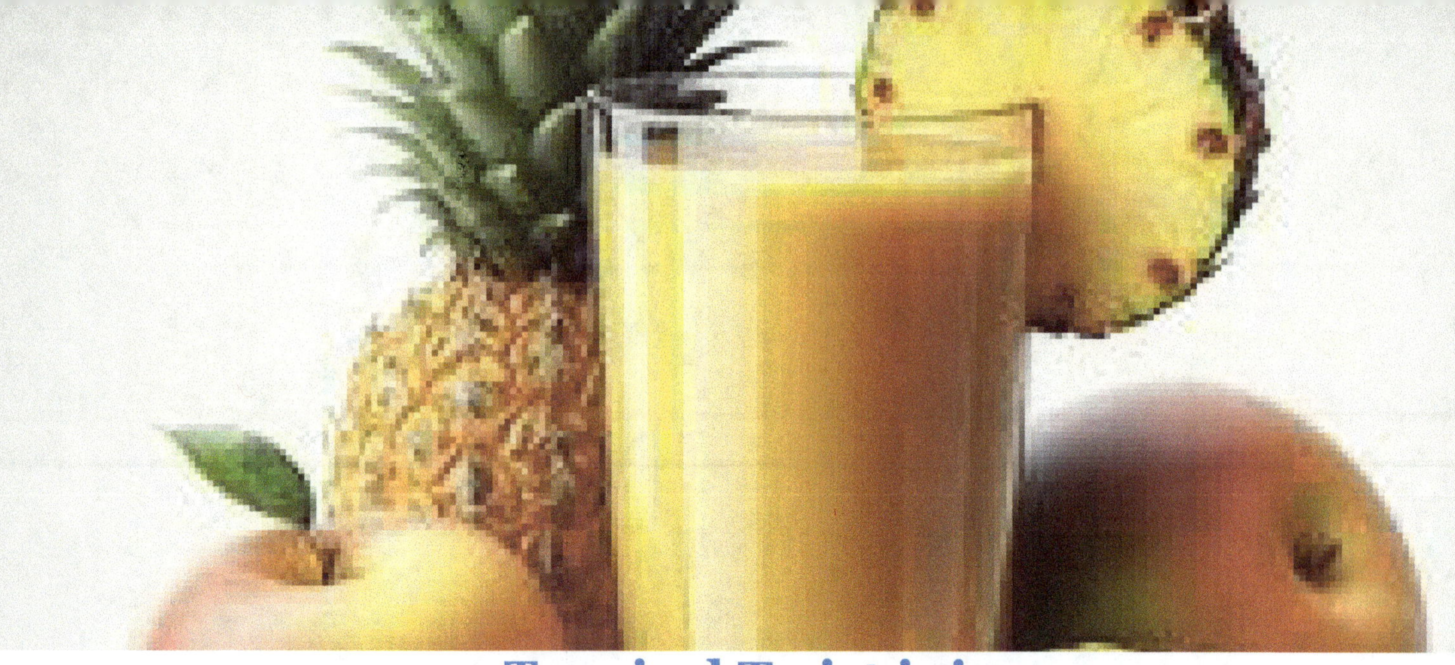

4. Tropical Twist juice

Introduction:

This juice is a delicious and refreshing way to start your day. The pineapple and mango provide sweetness and vitamins A and C, while the coconut water adds electrolytes.

Ingredients:

1 cup pineapple, peeled and diced

1 cup mango, peeled and diced

1 cup coconut water

Instructions:

Wash all of the ingredients well.

Cut the beet into small pieces.

Add all of the ingredients to a juicer and blend until smooth.

Serve immediately.

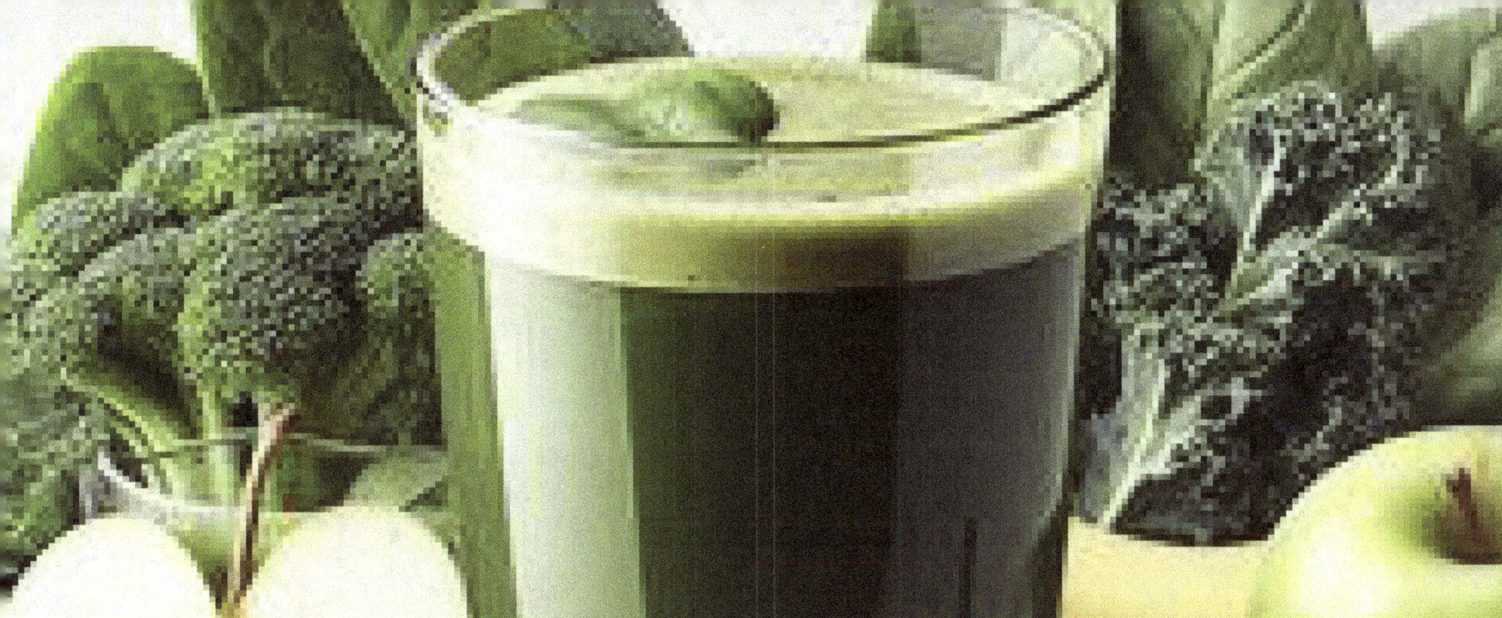

5. The Mighty Matcha Juice

Introduction:

This juice is a great way to start your day with a boost of energy and focus. The matcha powder provides caffeine and L-theanine, which improve alertness and concentration. The spinach and kale add vitamins and minerals, while the apple and banana add sweetness and creaminess.

Ingredients:

1 teaspoon matcha powder

1 cup spinach

1 cup kale

1 apple, peeled and cored

1 banana

1 cup almond milk

Instructions:

Wash all of the ingredients well.

Cut the apple and banana into small pieces.

Include Add all the ingredients to a blender and blend until smooth.

Serve immediately.

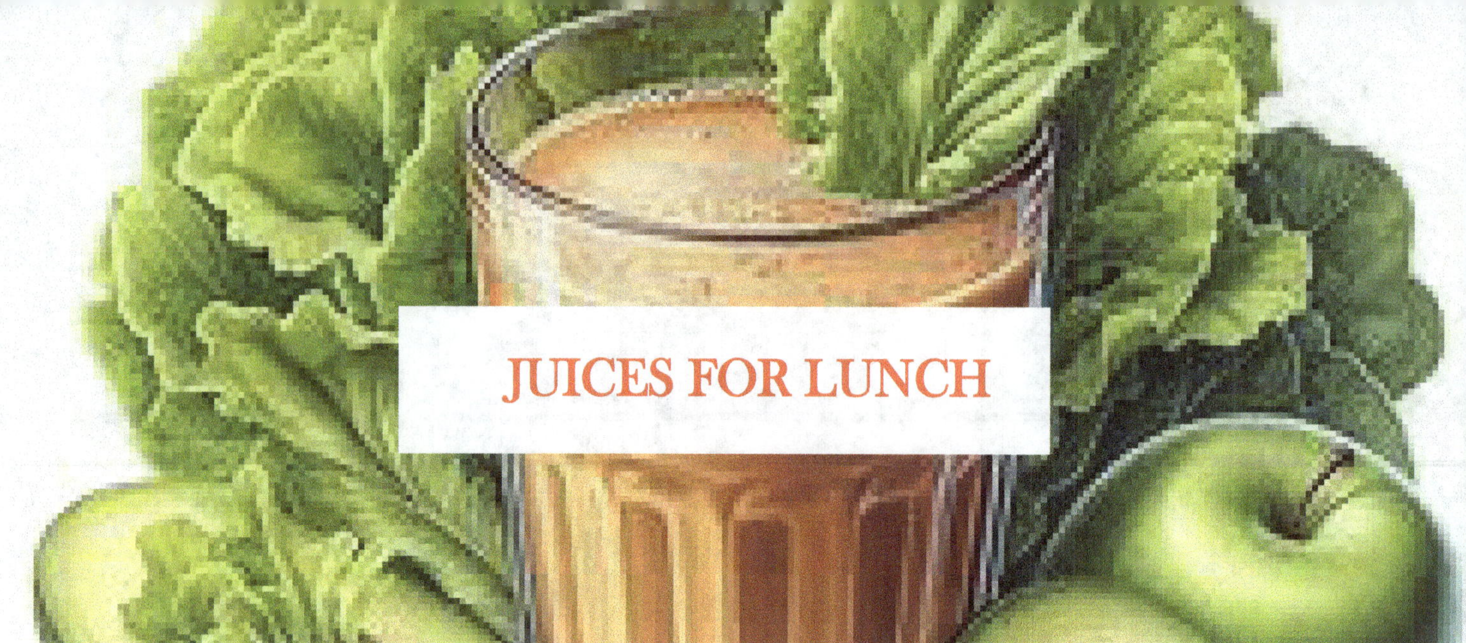

6. Hearty Healer juice

Introduction:

This juice is a hearty and filling meal perfect for lunch. The avocado and nuts provide healthy fats and protein, while the greens and vegetables add vitamins and minerals. This juice is also a good source of fiber, which can help you feel full and satisfied.

Ingredients:

1 avocado

1/2 cup nuts (any kind)

1 cup greens (spinach, kale, or romaine lettuce)

1/2 cup vegetables (carrots, cucumbers, or celery)

1 cup water

Instructions:

Wash all of the ingredients well.

Cut the avocado, nuts, and vegetables into small pieces.

Include all the ingredients in a blender and blend until smooth.

Serve immediately.

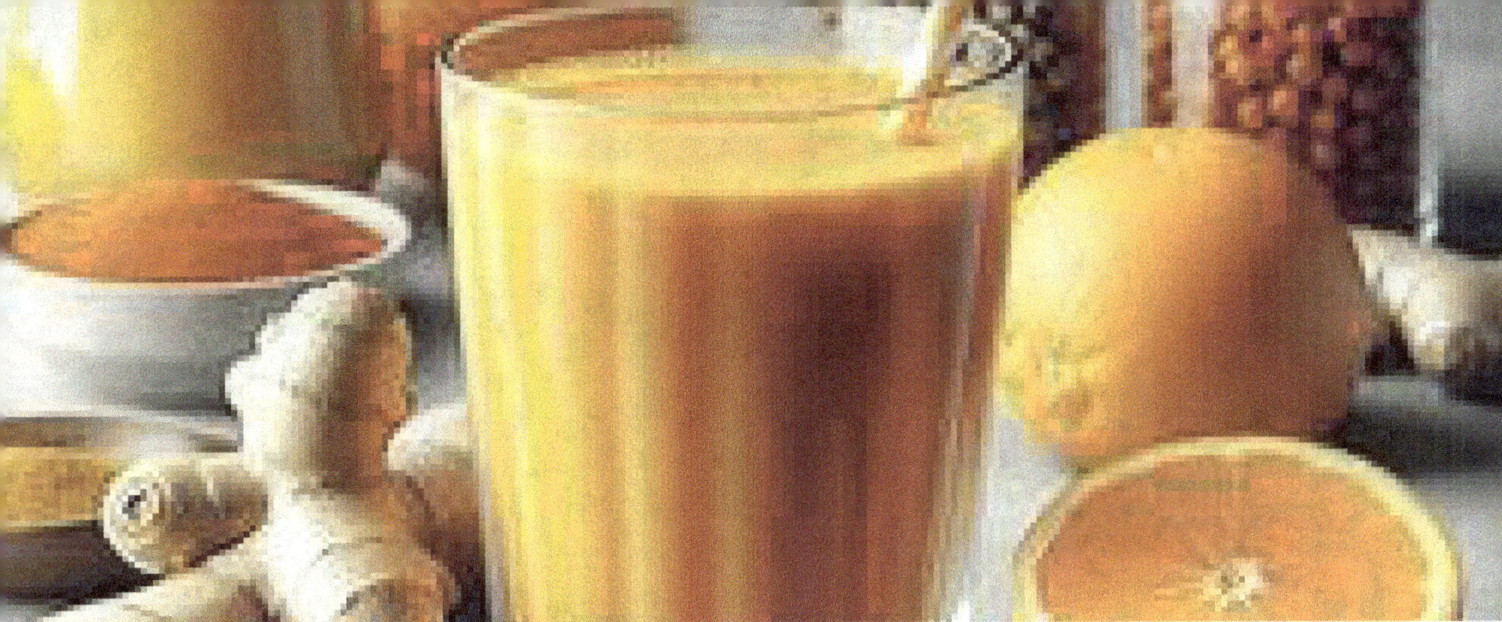

7. Spicy Immunity Booster juice

Introduction:

This juice contains vitamins and minerals that can help boost your immune system. The ginger, turmeric, and cayenne pepper have anti-inflammatory and antioxidant properties, while the carrots and oranges provide vitamins A and C. This juice is also a good source of potassium, which is essential for

Ingredients:

1/2 inch peeled and chopped ginger root

1/4 inch turmeric root, peeled and chopped

1/4 teaspoon cayenne pepper

1 cup carrots

1 orange, peeled and segmented

Instructions:

Wash all of the ingredients well.

Cut the carrots and orange into small pieces.

Add all of the ingredients to a juicer and blend until smooth.

Serve immediately.

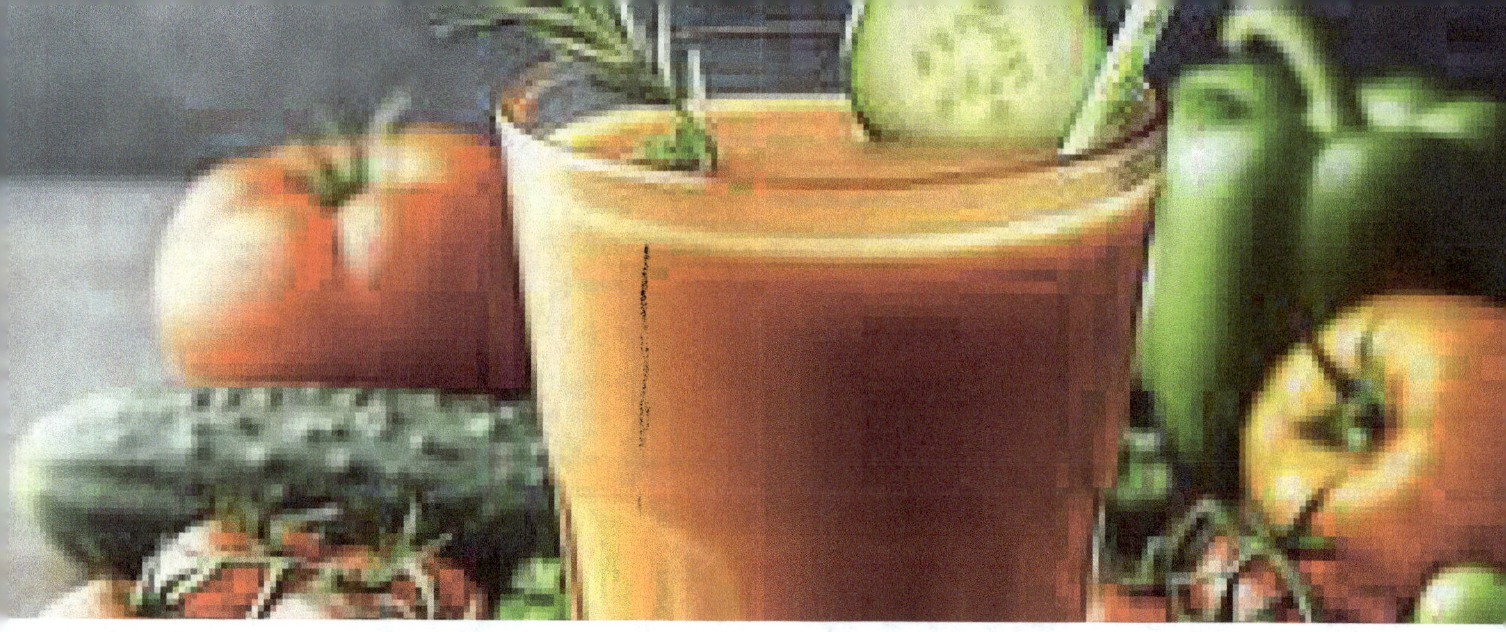

8. Mediterranean Medley juice

Introduction:

This juice is a tasty and delightful way of getting your daily dosage of vitamin C. The tomatoes, cucumbers, and bell peppers provide vitamins A and C, while the olive oil adds healthy fats. This juice is also a good source of potassium, which is necessary for blood pressure regulation.

Ingredients:

1 tomato, cored and sliced

1 cucumber, peeled and sliced

1/2 green bell pepper, cored and sliced

1 tablespoon olive oil

1/2 cup water

Instructions:

Wash all of the ingredients well.

Slice the tomato, cucumber, and bell pepper into small pieces.

Add all of the ingredients to a juicer and blend until smooth.

Serve immediately.

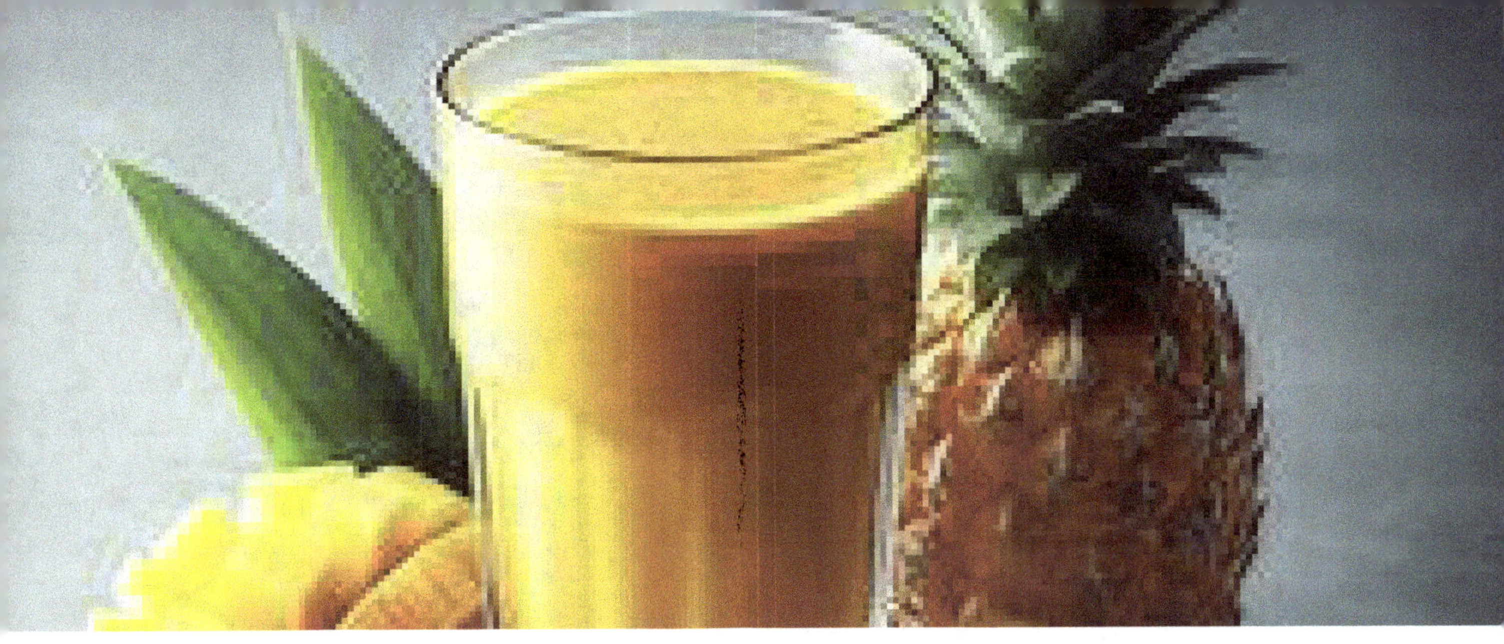

9. Tropical Turmeric Twist juice

Introduction:

This juice is a tasty and delightful way of getting your daily dosage of turmeric. The pineapple, mango, and coconut water provide sweetness and electrolytes, while the turmeric adds anti-inflammatory and antioxidant properties.

Ingredients:

1 cup pineapple, peeled and diced

1 cup mango, peeled and diced

1 cup coconut water

1/2 inch turmeric root, peeled and chopped

Instructions:

Wash all of the ingredients well.

Cut the pineapple and mango into small pieces.

Add all of the ingredients to a juicer and blend until smooth.

Serve immediately.

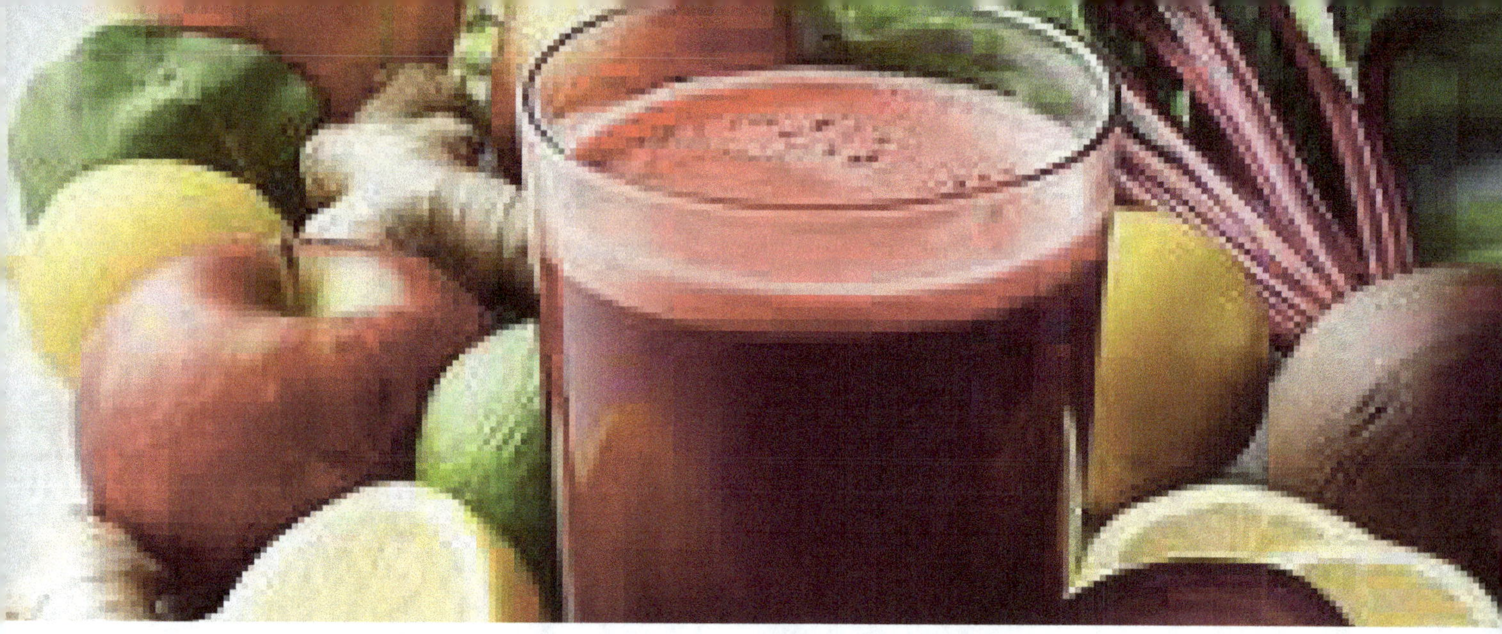

10. Beet Blast juice

Introduction:

This juice is a nutrient-rich power shot perfect for lunch. Beets are high in vitamins A and C, potassium, and iron. Both turmeric and ginger contain antioxidants and anti-inflammatory compounds, while apple and lemon add sweetness and tartness.

Ingredients:

1 beet, peeled and diced

1/2 inch peeled and chopped ginger root

1/4 inch turmeric root, peeled and chopped

1 apple, peeled and cored

1/2 lemon, peeled and juiced

Instructions:

Wash all of the ingredients well.

Cut the beet, apple, and ginger into small pieces.

Add all of the ingredients to a juicer and blend until smooth.

Serve immediately.

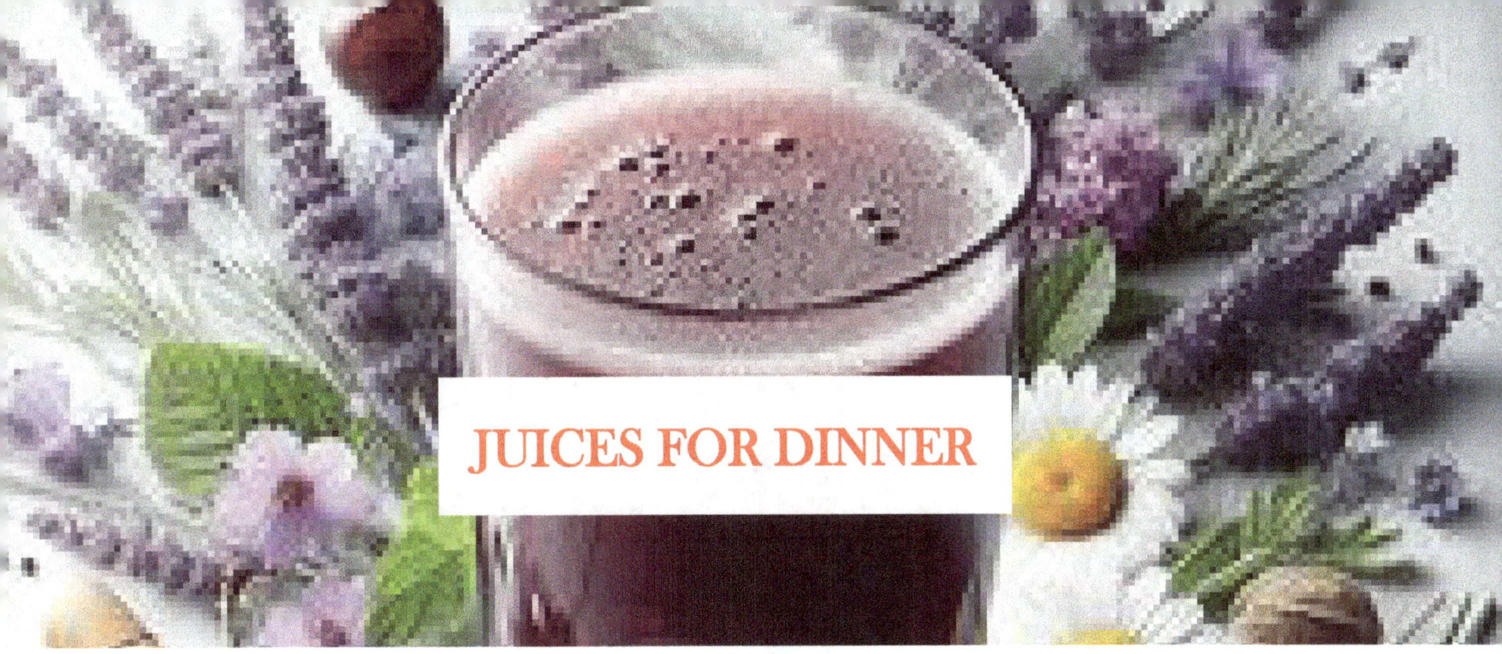

11. The Evening Elixir Juice

Introduction:

This juice is a delicious and nutritious way to end your day. It's rich in minerals, vitamins, and antioxidants that can help you relax and unwind. The tart cherry juice contains melatonin, which might help you sleep better. The lavender and chamomile are calming, while the rose water adds a delicate floral flavor.

Ingredients:

1 cup tart cherry juice

1/2 cup water

1/4 teaspoon lavender flowers

1/4 teaspoon chamomile flowers

1 tablespoon rose water

Instructions:

Wash all of the ingredients well.

Include all the ingredients in a blender and blend until smooth.

Serve immediately.

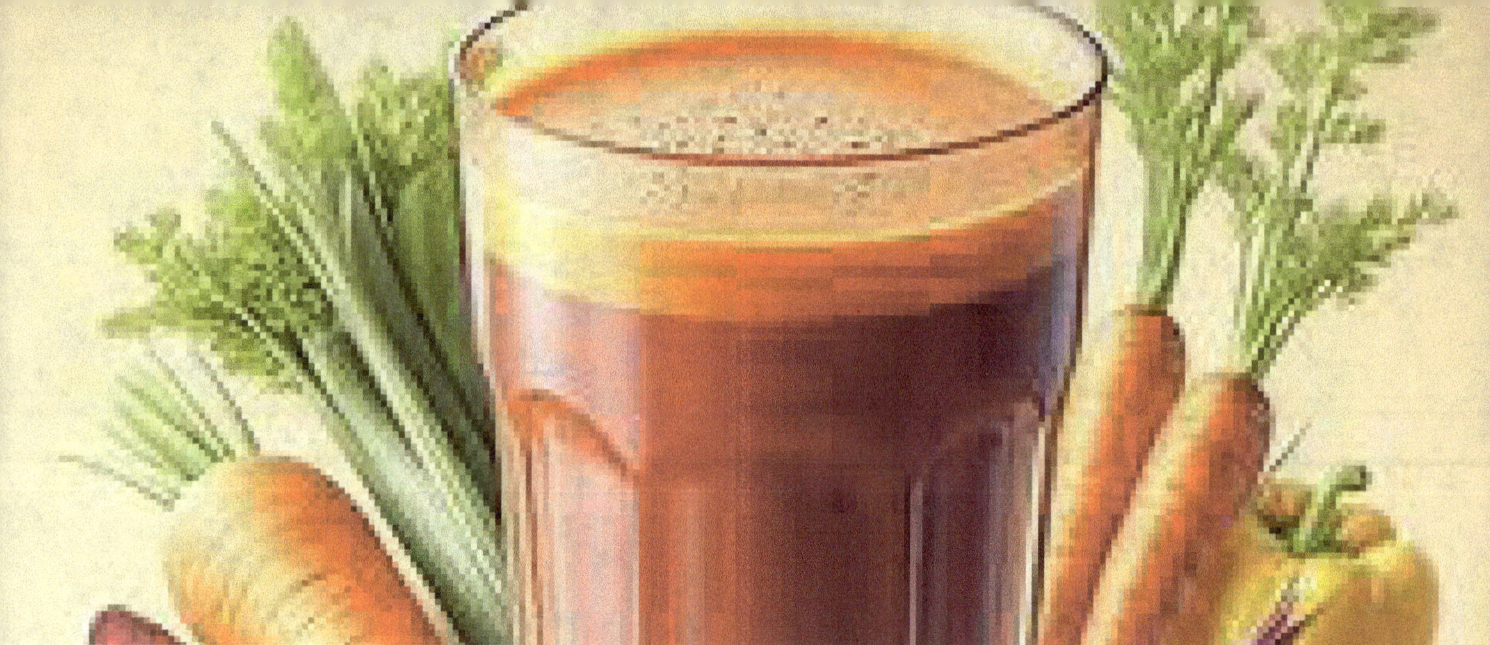

12. The Spicy Sunset Juice

Introduction:

This juice is a flavorful and fiery way to end your day. The carrots, beets, and ginger provide vitamins A and C, while the cayenne pepper adds a kick of heat. The turmeric and black pepper enhance the absorption of the turmeric's anti-inflammatory properties.

Ingredients:

1 cup carrots, diced

1 beet, diced

1/2 inch and chopped ginger root

1/4 teaspoon cayenne pepper

1/4 teaspoon turmeric powder

1/4 teaspoon black pepper

Instructions:

Wash all of the ingredients well.

Cut the beet into small pieces.

Add all of the ingredients to a juicer and blend until smooth.

Serve immediately.

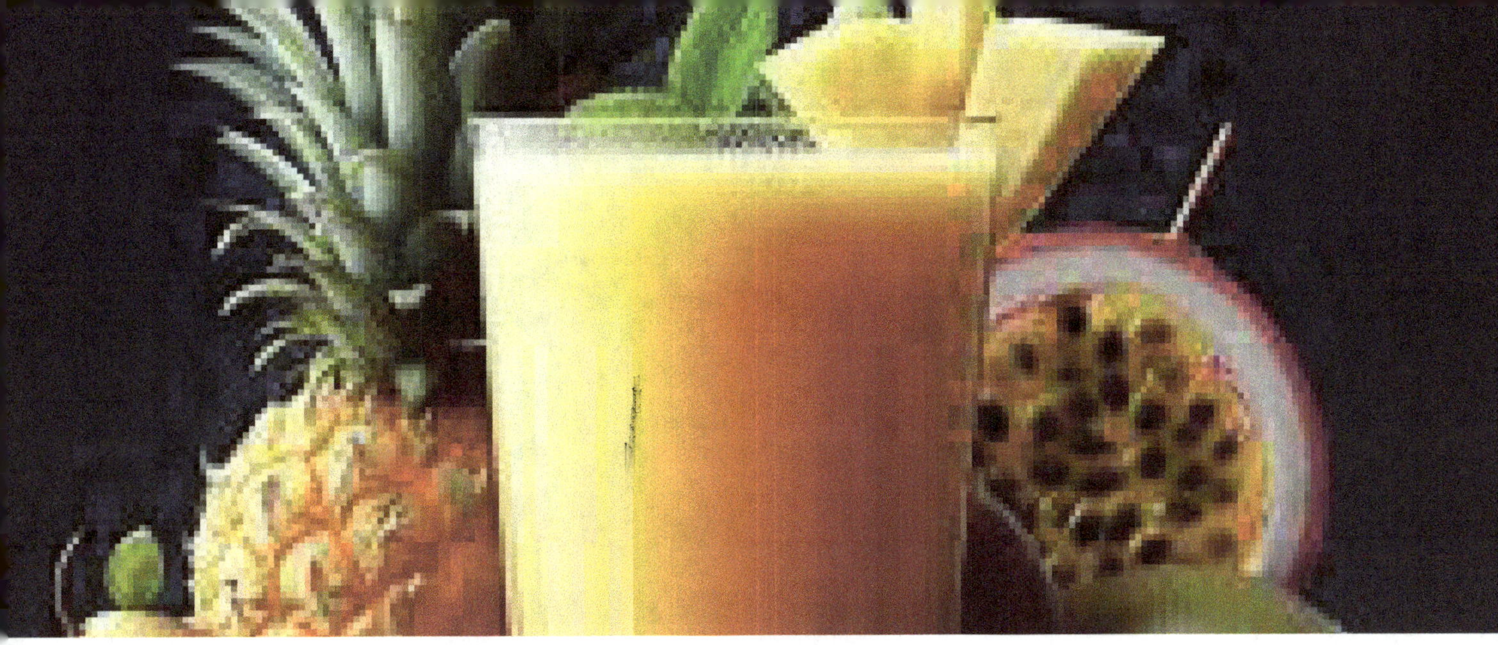

13. The Tropical Twilight Juice

Introduction:

This juice is a sweet and refreshing way to end your day. The pineapple, mango, and coconut water provide vitamins A and C and electrolytes. The passion fruit and guava add a tart and exotic flavor.

Ingredients:

1 cup pineapple, diced

1 cup mango, diced

1 cup coconut water

1 passion fruit, halved and scooped

1/2 guava, peeled and seeded

Instructions:

Wash all of the ingredients well.

Cut the pineapple, mango, passion fruit, and guava into small pieces.

Add all of the ingredients to a juicer and blend until smooth.

Serve immediately.

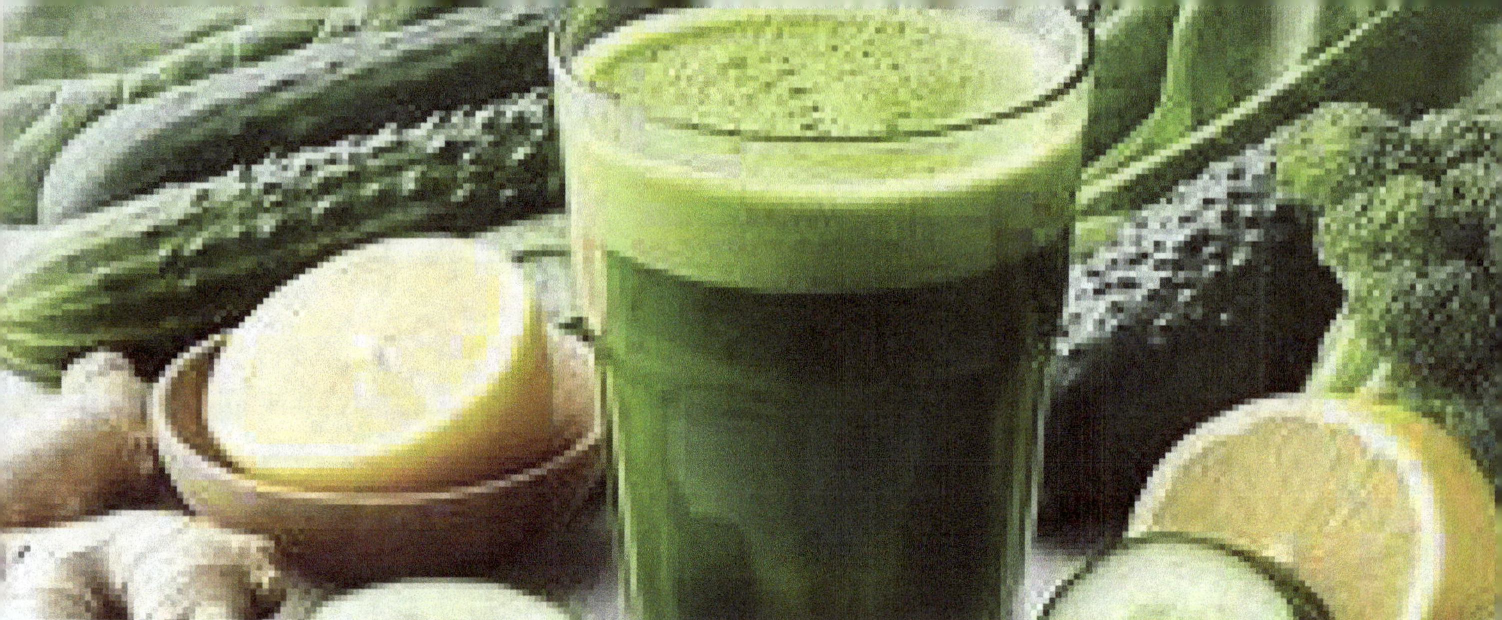

14. The Green Goddess Juice

Introduction:

This juice is a nutrient-rich powerhouse perfect for dinner. The kale, spinach, and celery provide vitamins A, C, and K, while the lemon and apple add sweetness and tartness. The cucumber and ginger add a refreshing and cleansing effect.

Ingredients:

1 cup kale

1 cup spinach

1/2 cup celery, chopped

1 lemon, peeled and juiced

1 apple, peeled and cored

1 cucumber, peeled and diced

1/2 inch peeled and chopped ginger root

Instructions:

Wash all of the ingredients well.

Cut the apple and cucumber into small pieces.

Add all of the ingredients to a juicer and blend until smooth.

Serve immediately.

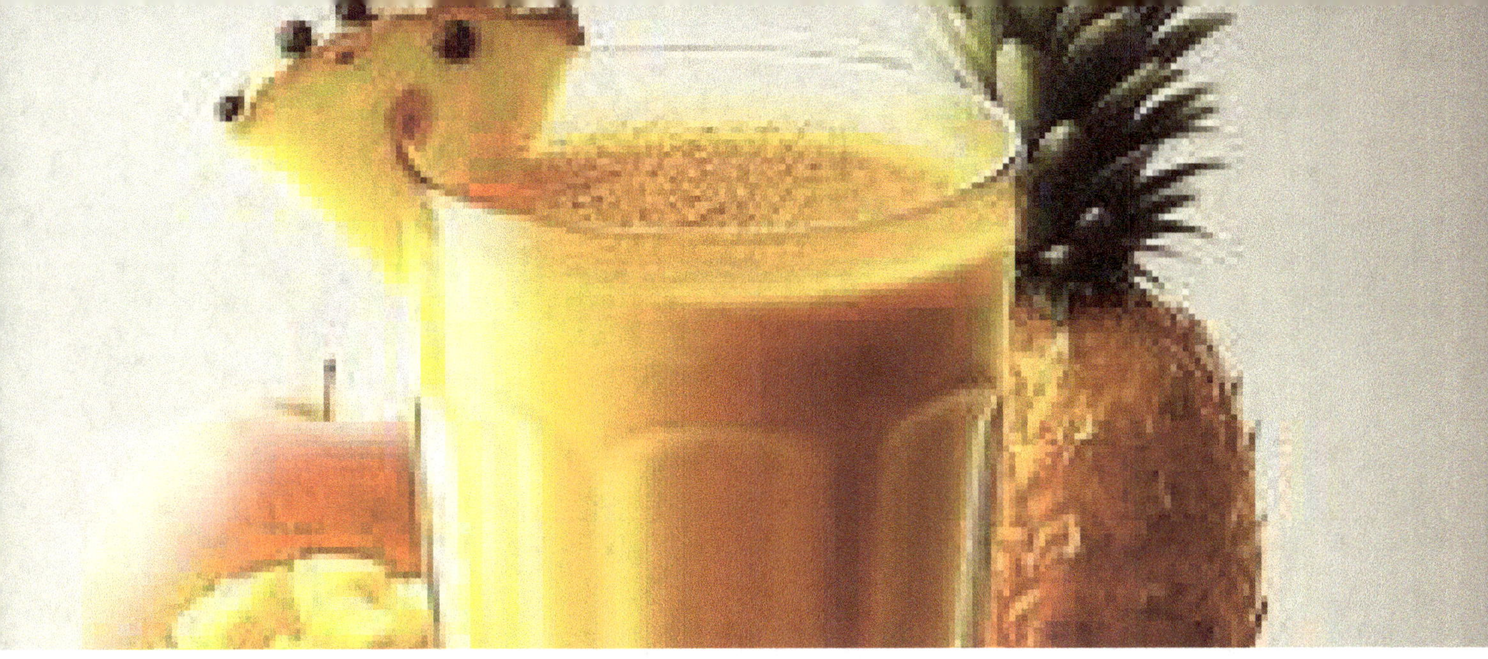

15. Golden Glow juice

Introduction:

This juice is packed with antioxidants and anti-inflammatory properties, making it a perfect way to end your day. The turmeric, ginger, and black pepper work together to boost the absorption of the turmeric's curcumin, a powerful antioxidant. The pineapple and mango add sweetness and tropical flavor, while the coconut water adds electrolytes.

Ingredients:

1/2 inch turmeric root, peeled and chopped

1/2 inch peeled and chopped ginger root

1/4 teaspoon black pepper

1 cup pineapple, diced

1 cup mango, diced

1 cup coconut water

Instructions:

Wash all of the ingredients well.

Cut the pineapple and mango into small pieces.

Add all of the ingredients to a juicer and blend until smooth.

Serve immediately.

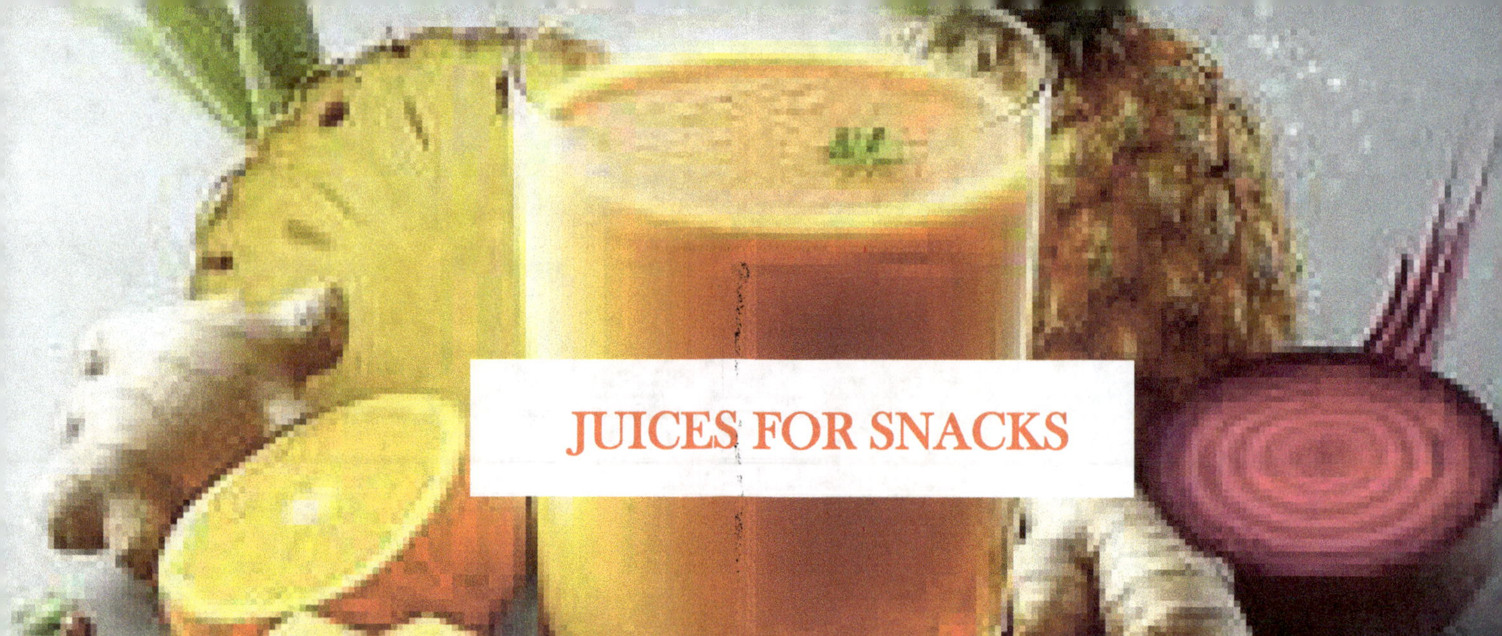

16. The Energy Boost Juice

Introduction:

This juice contains vitamins, minerals, and antioxidants to help you power through your afternoon. The carrots and beets provide vitamins A and C, while the ginger and turmeric have anti-inflammatory and antioxidant properties. The pineapple and orange add sweetness and citrus flavor.

Ingredients:

1 cup carrots, diced

1 beet, diced

1/2 inch peeled and chopped ginger root

1/4 inch turmeric root, peeled and chopped

1 cup pineapple, diced

1 orange, peeled and segmented

Instructions:

Wash all of the ingredients well.

Cut the carrots, beets, pineapple, and orange into small pieces.

Add all of the ingredients to a juicer and blend until smooth.

Serve immediately.

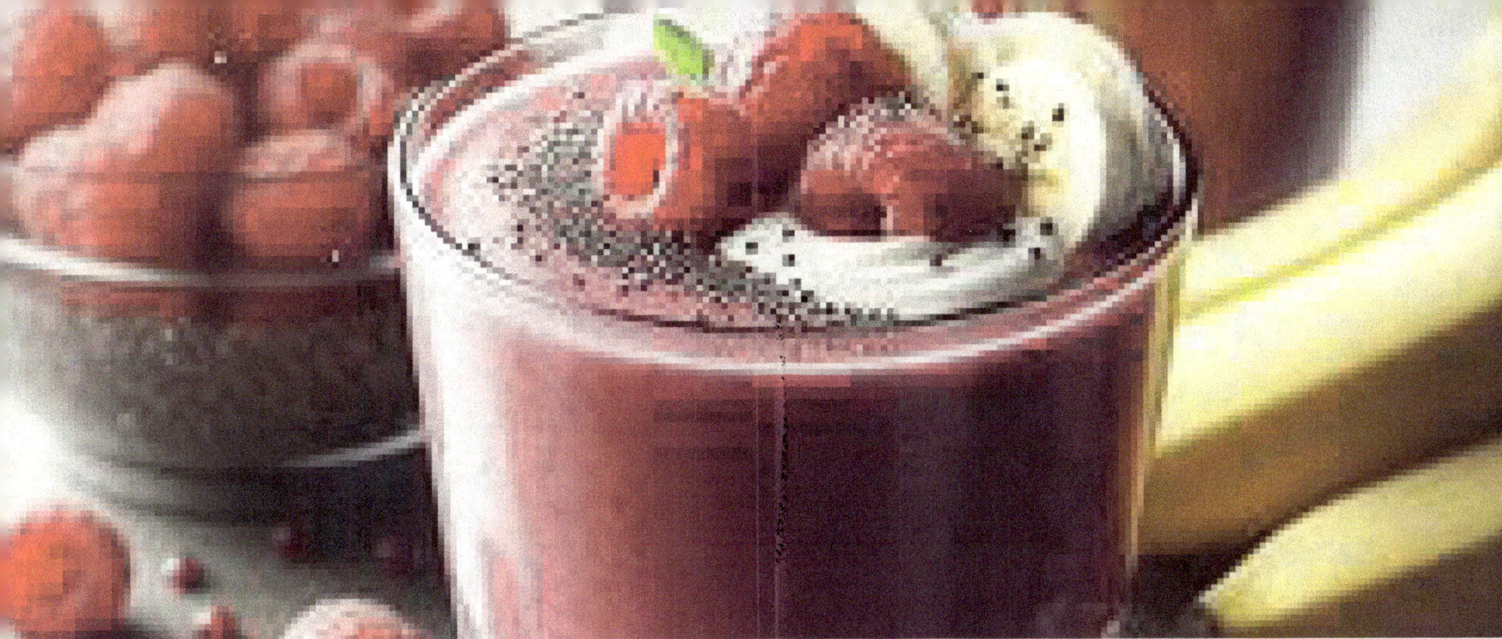

17. The Berry Bliss Juice

Introduction:

This juice is a sweet, satisfying snack with antioxidants and vitamins. The berries provide vitamins A and C, while the banana and yogurt add sweetness and creaminess. The chia seeds add fiber and protein, making this juice a balanced and filling snack.

Ingredients:

1 cup berries (any kind)

1 banana, peeled and sliced

1/2 cup yogurt (plain or Greek)

1 tablespoon chia seeds

1/2 cup water

Instructions:

Wash all of the ingredients well.

Include all of the ingredients in a blender and blend until smooth.

Serve immediately.

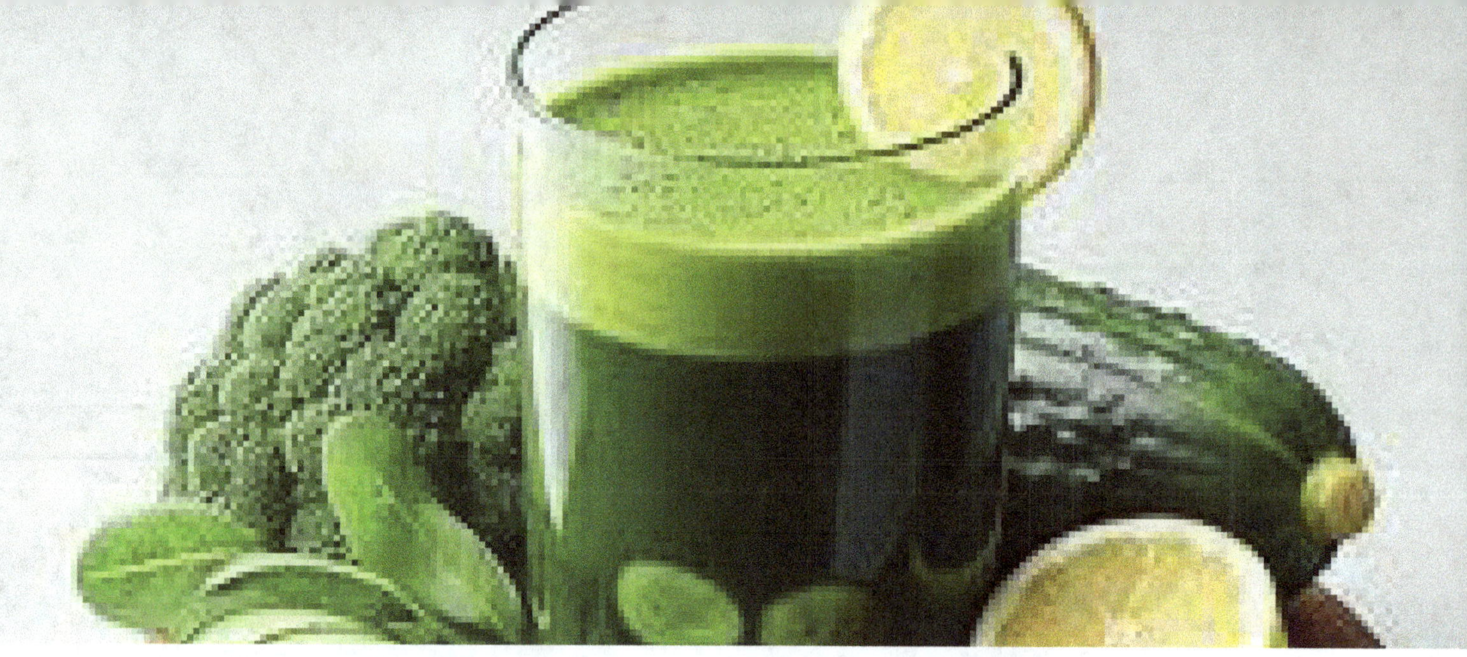

18. Green Powerhouse juice

Introduction:

This juice is a nutrient-rich powerhouse perfect for a snack. The leafy greens provide vitamins A, C, and K, while the celery and cucumber add hydration and electrolytes. The lemon and ginger add a refreshing and cleansing effect.

Ingredients:

1 cup leafy greens (spinach, kale, or romaine lettuce)

1/2 cup celery, chopped

1/2 cucumber, peeled and diced

1 lemon, peeled and juiced

1/2 inch peeled and chopped ginger root

Instructions:

Wash all of the ingredients well.

Cut the cucumber into small pieces.

Add all of the ingredients to a juicer and blend until smooth.

Serve immediately.

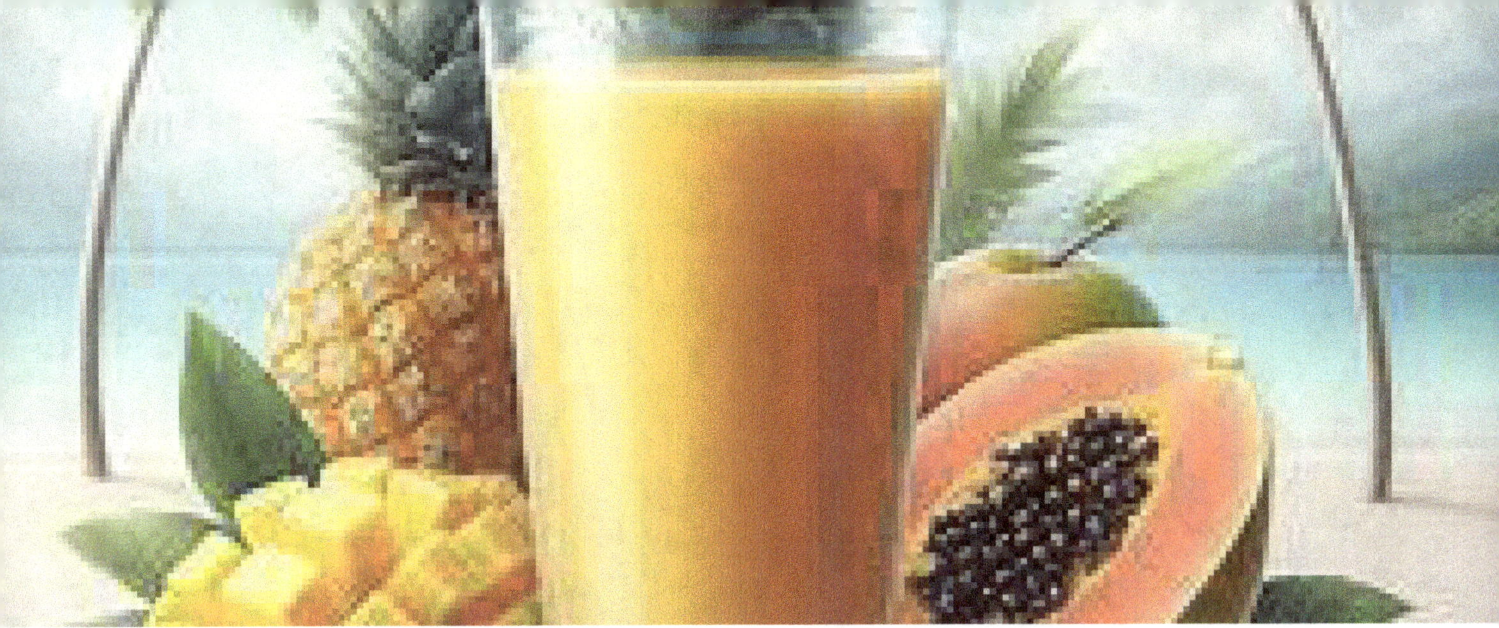

19. The Tropical Escape Juice

Introduction:

This juice is a delicious, refreshing snack that will transport you to your tropical oasis. The pineapple, mango, and coconut water provide vitamins A and C and electrolytes. The papaya and guava add a sweet and exotic flavor.

Ingredients:

1 cup pineapple, diced

1 cup mango, diced

1 cup coconut water

1 papaya, peeled and seeded

1/2 guava, peeled and seeded

Instructions:

Wash all of the ingredients well.

Cut the pineapple, mango, papaya, and guava into small pieces.

Add all of the ingredients to a juicer and blend until smooth.

Serve immediately.

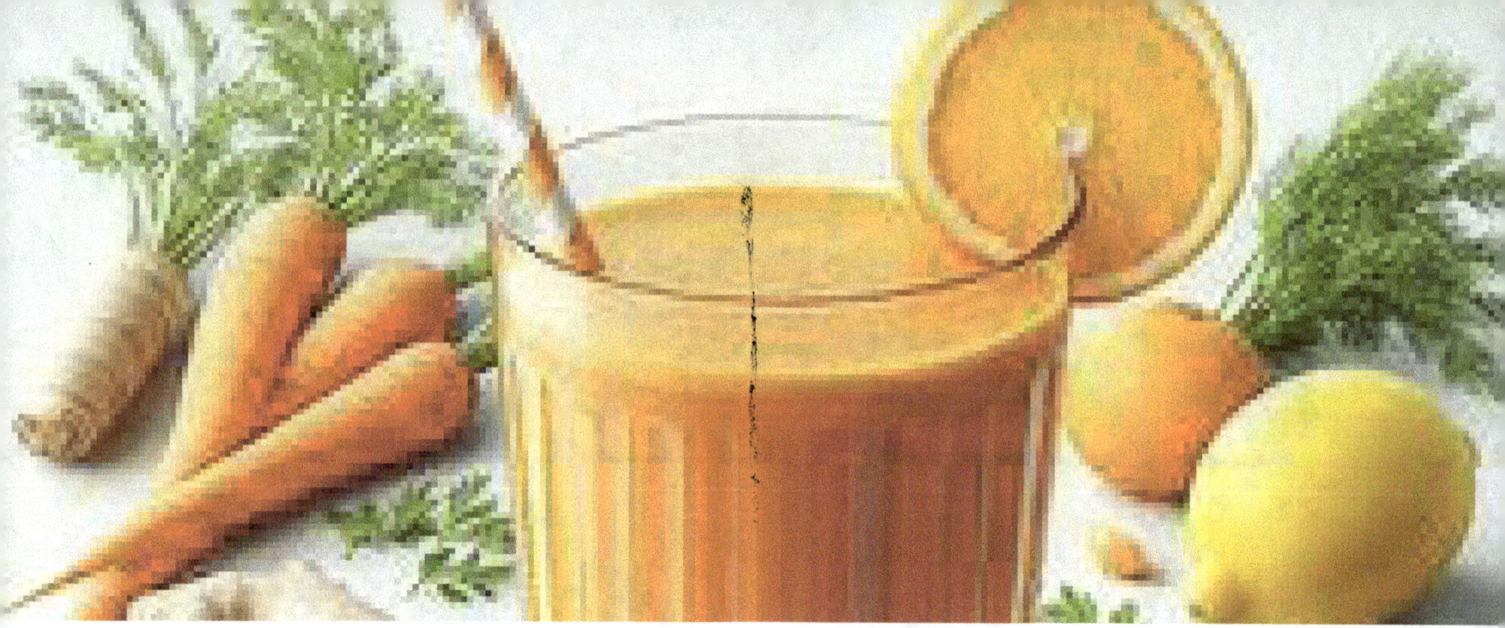

20. The Immunity Boost Juice

Introduction:

This juice contains minerals, vitamins, and antioxidants that can assist in boosting your immune system. The carrots, oranges, and ginger provide vitamins A and C, while the turmeric and black pepper have anti-inflammatory and antioxidant properties. The lemon and cayenne pepper add a kick of flavor and heat.

Ingredients:

1 cup carrots, diced

1 orange, peeled and segmented

1/2 inch peeled and chopped ginger root

1/4 inch turmeric root, peeled and chopped

1/4 teaspoon black pepper

1/2 lemon, juiced

1/4 teaspoon cayenne pepper

Instructions:

Wash all of the ingredients well.

Cut the carrots and orange into small pieces.

Add all of the ingredients to a juicer and blend until smooth.

Serve immediately.

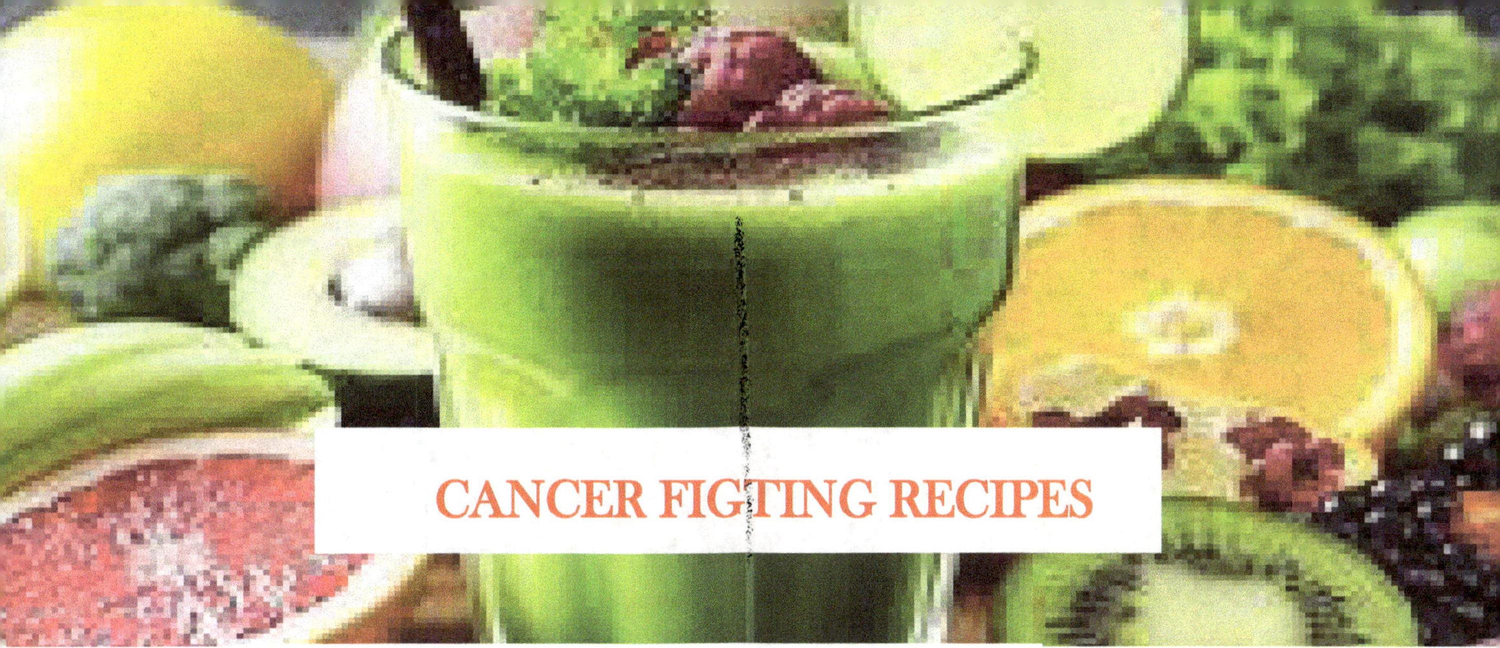

21. The Cancer-Fighter Juice

Introduction:

This juice is packed with cancer-fighting compounds from fruits and vegetables like berries, broccoli, and turmeric. It's also a good source of vitamins and minerals that can help to support the immune system.

Ingredients:

1 cup blueberries

1 cup raspberries

1/2 cup broccoli florets

1/4 cup turmeric root, peeled and chopped

1/4 cup ginger root, peeled and chopped

1/2 lemon, peeled and juiced

Instructions:

1. Wash all of the ingredients well.

2. Cut the broccoli and turmeric into small pieces.

3. Add all of the ingredients to a juicer and blend until smooth.

Serve immediately.

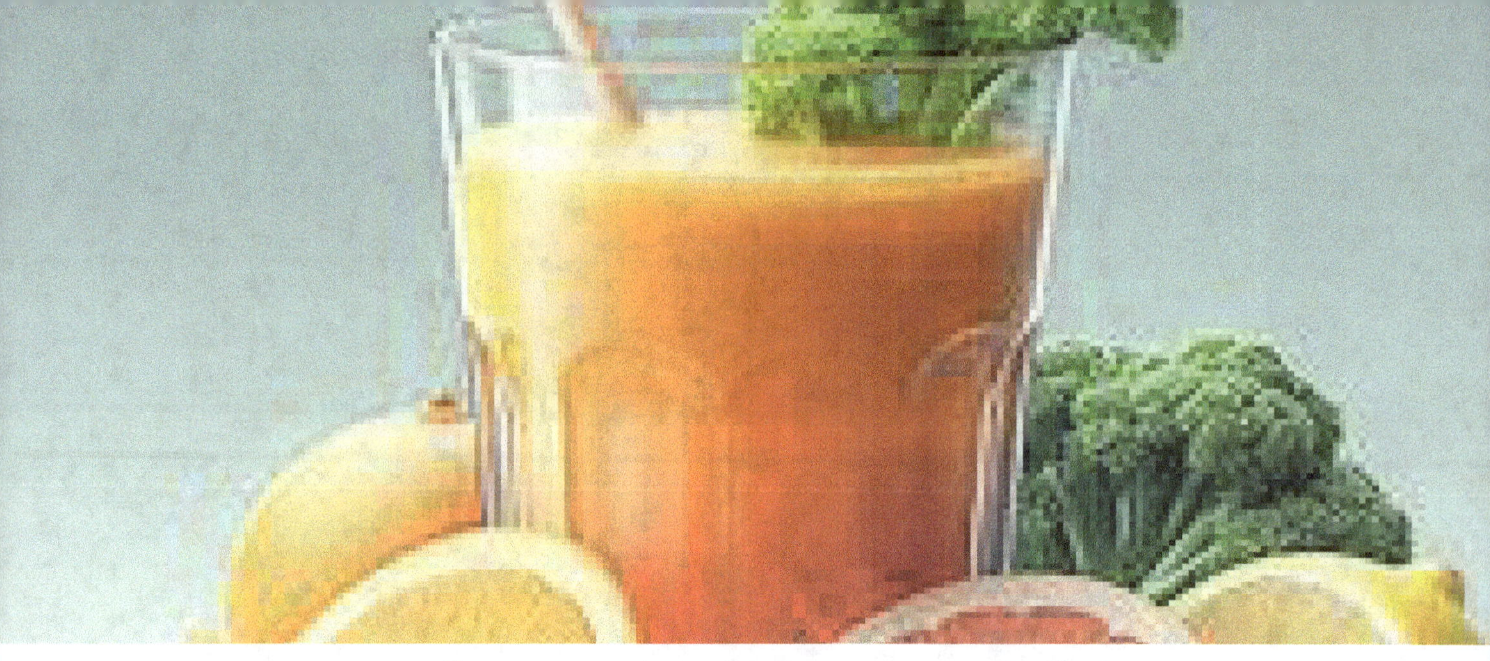

22. The Immune Booster Juice

Introduction:

This juice is prepared to boost your immune system with citrus fruits, leafy greens, and carrots. It's also a good source of antioxidants, which can help to fight off damage from free radicals.

Ingredients:

1 orange, peeled and juiced

1 grapefruit, peeled and juiced

1 lemon, peeled and juiced

1 cup kale

1 cup carrots

Instructions:

Wash all of the ingredients well.

Cut the kale and carrots into small pieces.

Add all of the ingredients to a juicer and blend until smooth.

Serve immediately.

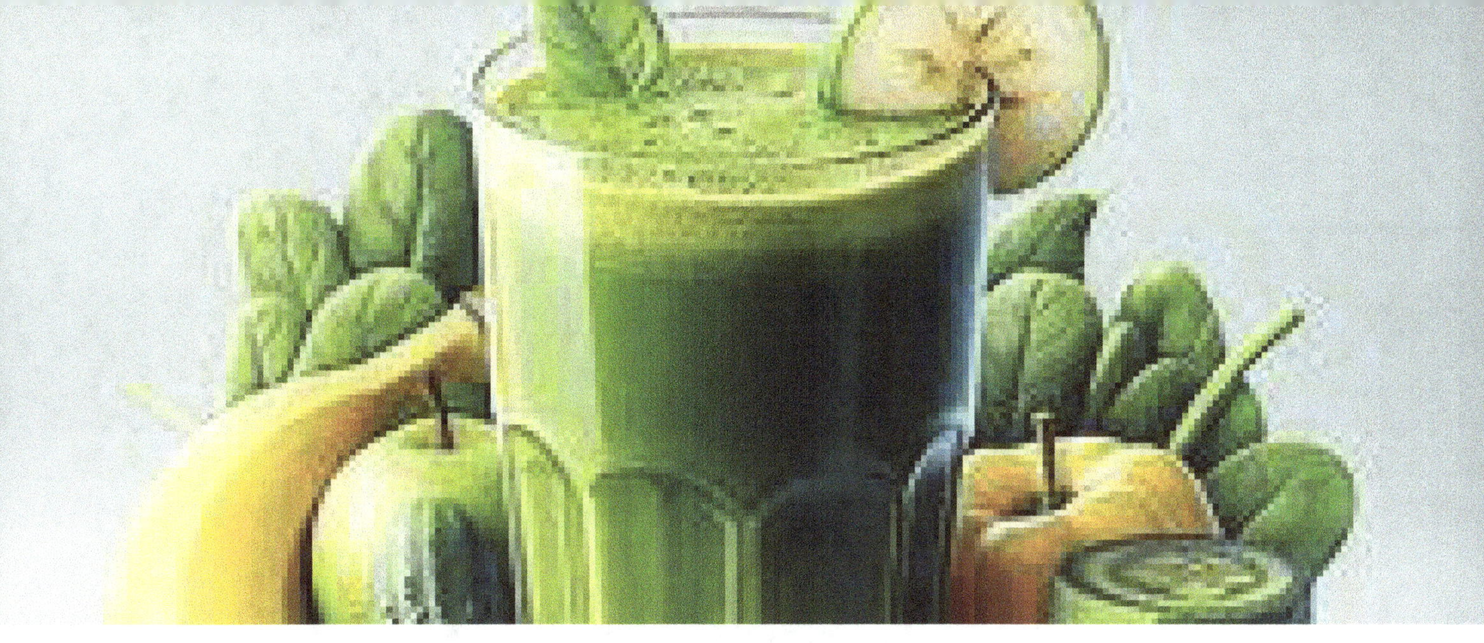

23. The Energy Booster Juice

Introduction:

This juice contains nutrients that can help boost your energy levels, including fruits like apples and bananas and vegetables like spinach and cucumber. It's also a good source of electrolytes, which can help to keep you hydrated.

Ingredients:

1 apple, peeled and cored

1 banana, peeled

1 cup spinach

1/2 cucumber, peeled and seeded

Instructions:

Wash all of the ingredients well.

Cut the apple and cucumber into small pieces.

Add all of the ingredients to a juicer and blend until smooth.

Serve immediately.

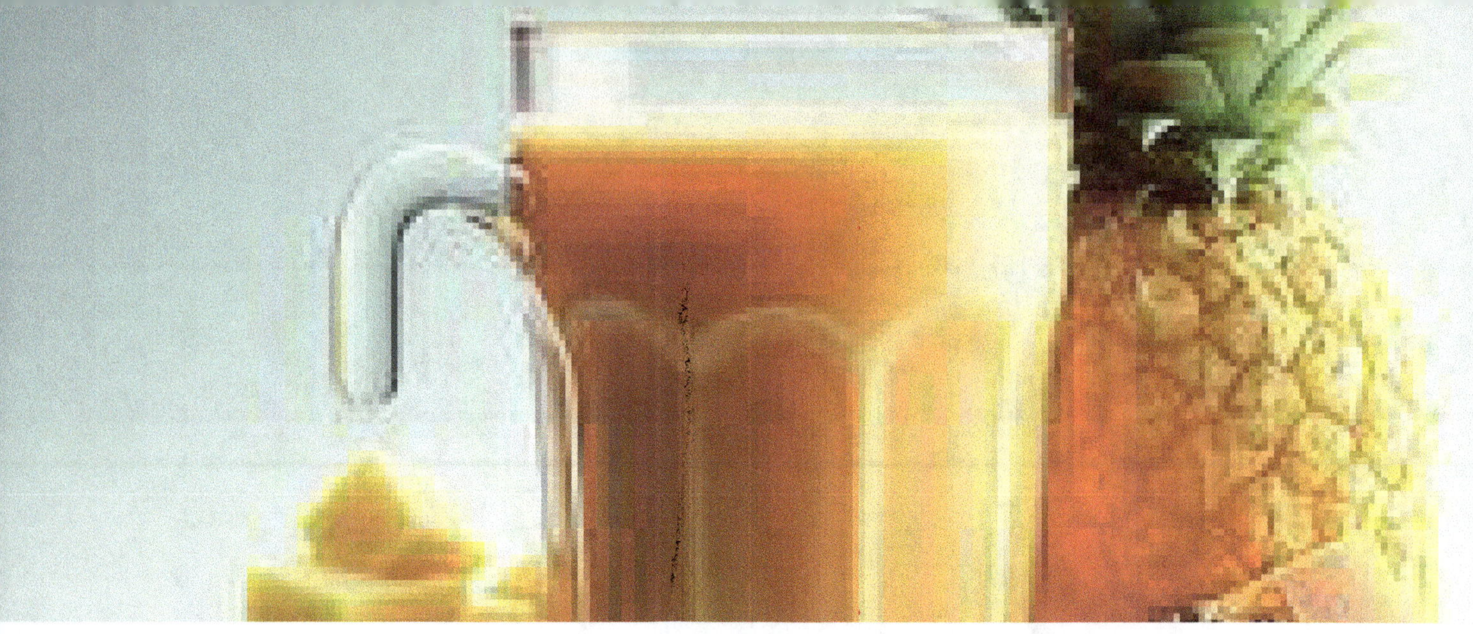

24. The Digestive Booster Juice

Introduction:

This juice is created to help digestion with ingredients like pineapple, papaya, and celery. It's also high in fiber, which can help keep the digestive tract healthy.

Ingredients:

1 cup pineapple, peeled and cored

1/2 papaya, peeled and seeded

2 celery stalks, cut into pieces

Instructions:

Wash all of the ingredients well.

Cut the pineapple and papaya into small pieces.

Add all of the ingredients to a juicer and blend until smooth.

Serve immediately.

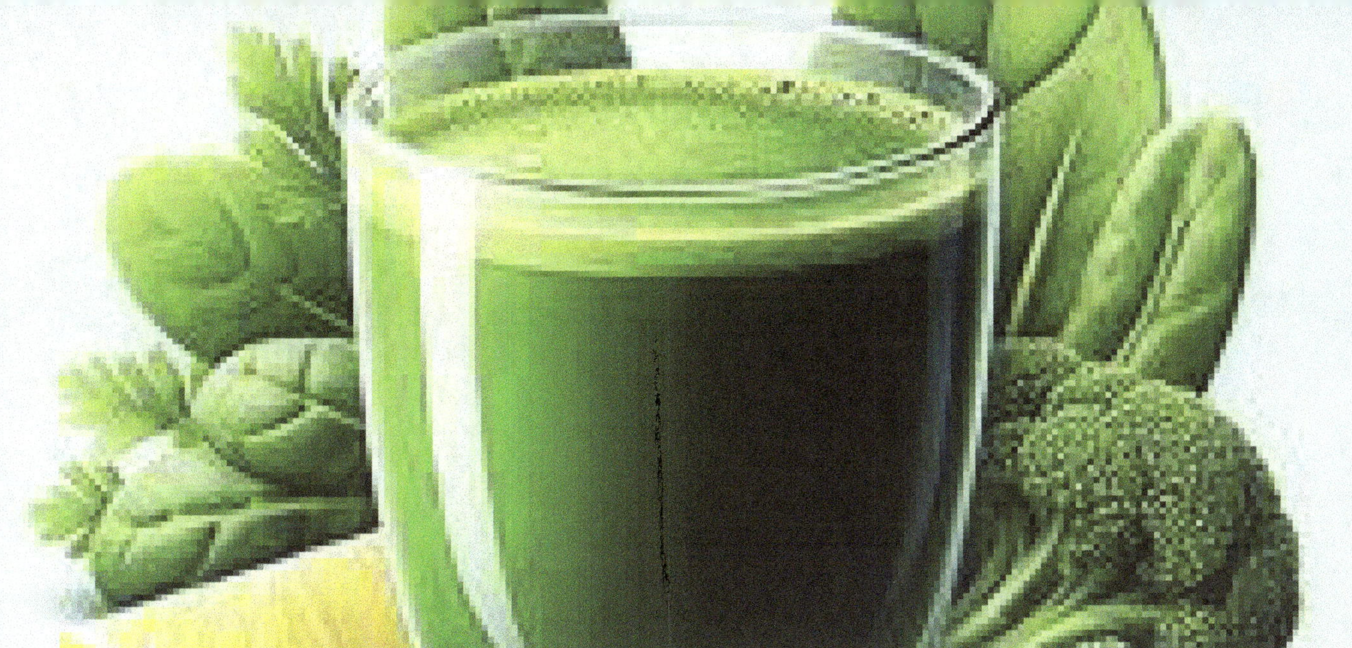

25. Green Broccoli and Apple Zest

Introduction:

This green juice is a delightful combination of broccoli and apple, providing a burst of flavor along with essential nutrients.

Ingredients:

1 cup of broccoli florets

1 green apple

1 cucumber

1/2 lemon, peeled

A handful of basil leaves

Instructions:

Wash all of the ingredients well.

Cut the green apple into small pieces.

Add all of the ingredients to a juicer and blend until smooth.

Garnish with basil leaves.

Serve immediately.

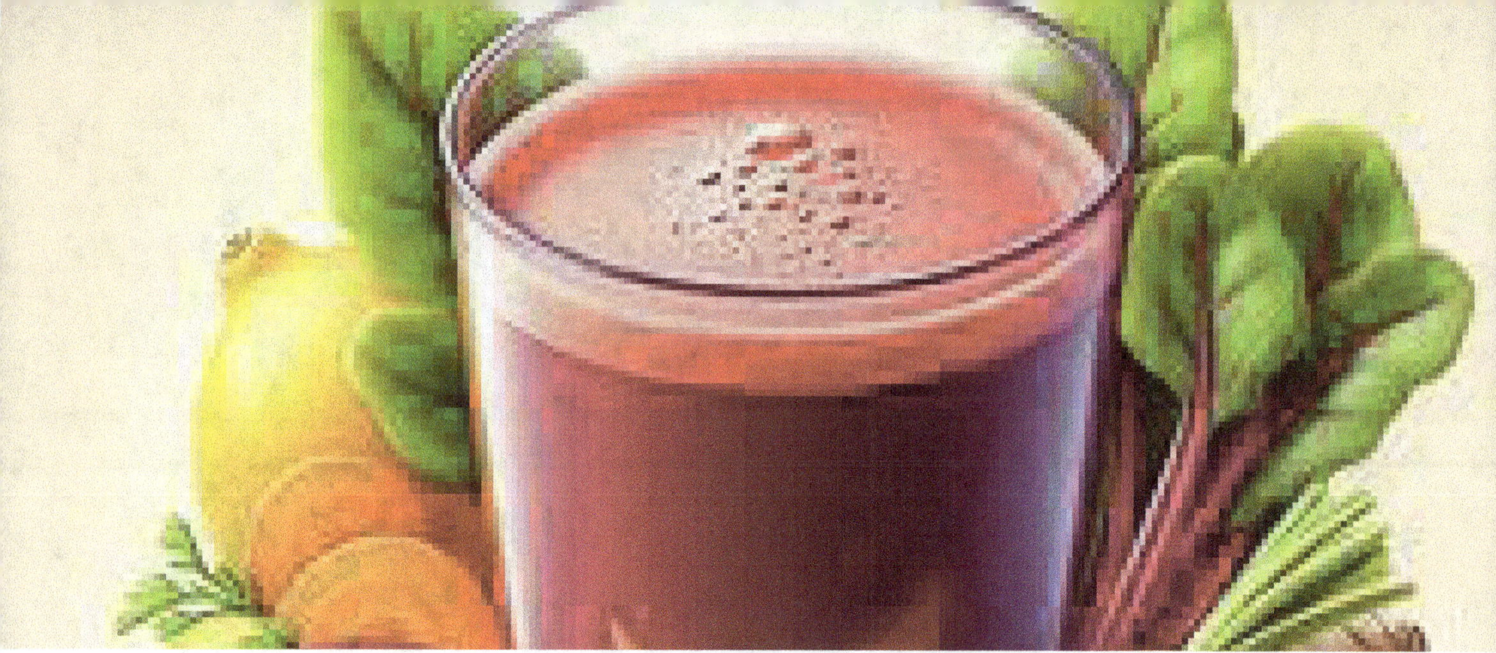

26. The Liver Detoxifier Juice

Introduction:

This juice is designed to help detoxify the liver, an essential organ for removing toxins from the body. The ingredients in this juice, including beets, carrots, and turmeric, are all known to support liver health.

Ingredients:

1 beet, peeled and quartered

2 carrots

1/2 inch turmeric root, peeled and chopped

1/4 cup lemon juice

Instructions:

Wash all of the ingredients well.

Cut the beet and carrots into small pieces.

Add all of the ingredients to a juicer and blend until smooth.

Serve immediately.

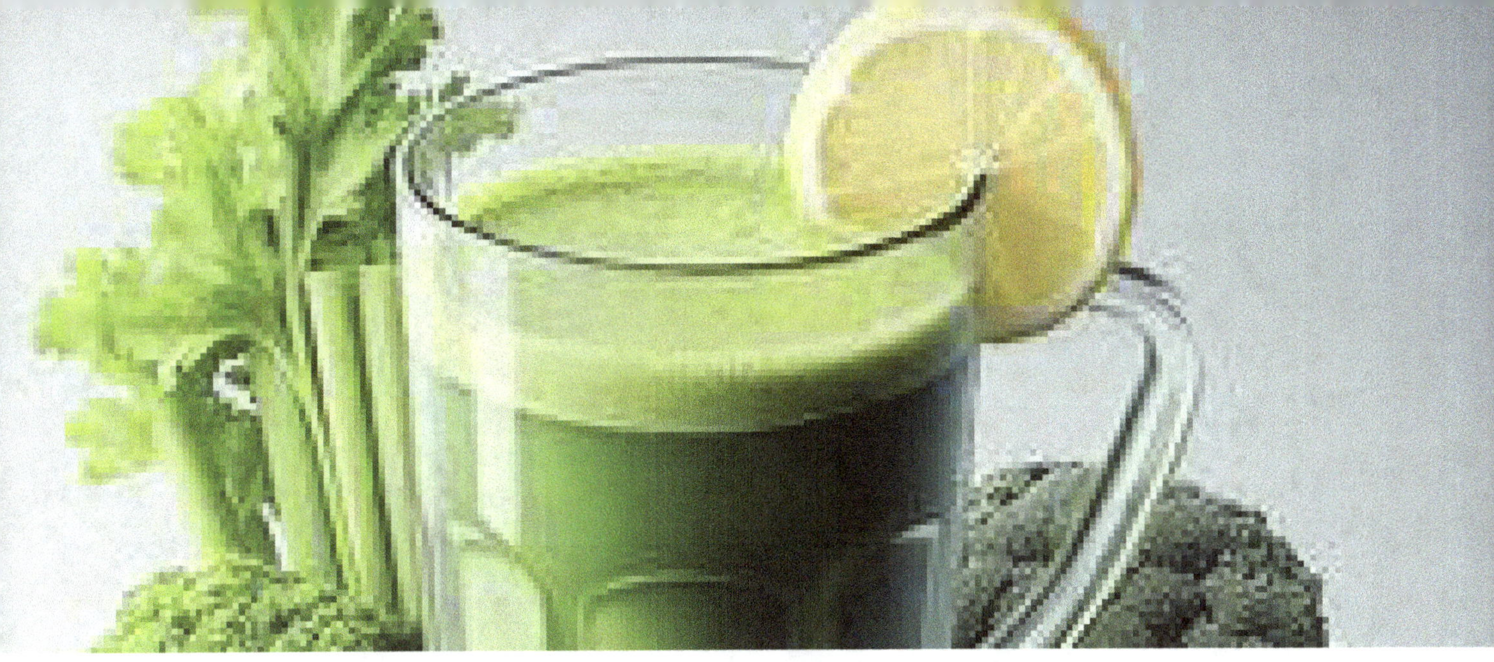

27. The Colon Cleanser Juice

Introduction:

This juice is created to help cleanse the colon and remove toxins from the body. The ingredients in this juice, including kale, cucumber, and celery, are all known to be beneficial for colon health.

Ingredients:

1 cup kale

1/2 cucumber, peeled and seeded

2 celery stalks, cut into pieces

Instructions:

Wash all of the ingredients well.

Cut the kale and cucumber into small pieces.

Add all of the ingredients to a juicer and blend until smooth.

Serve immediately.

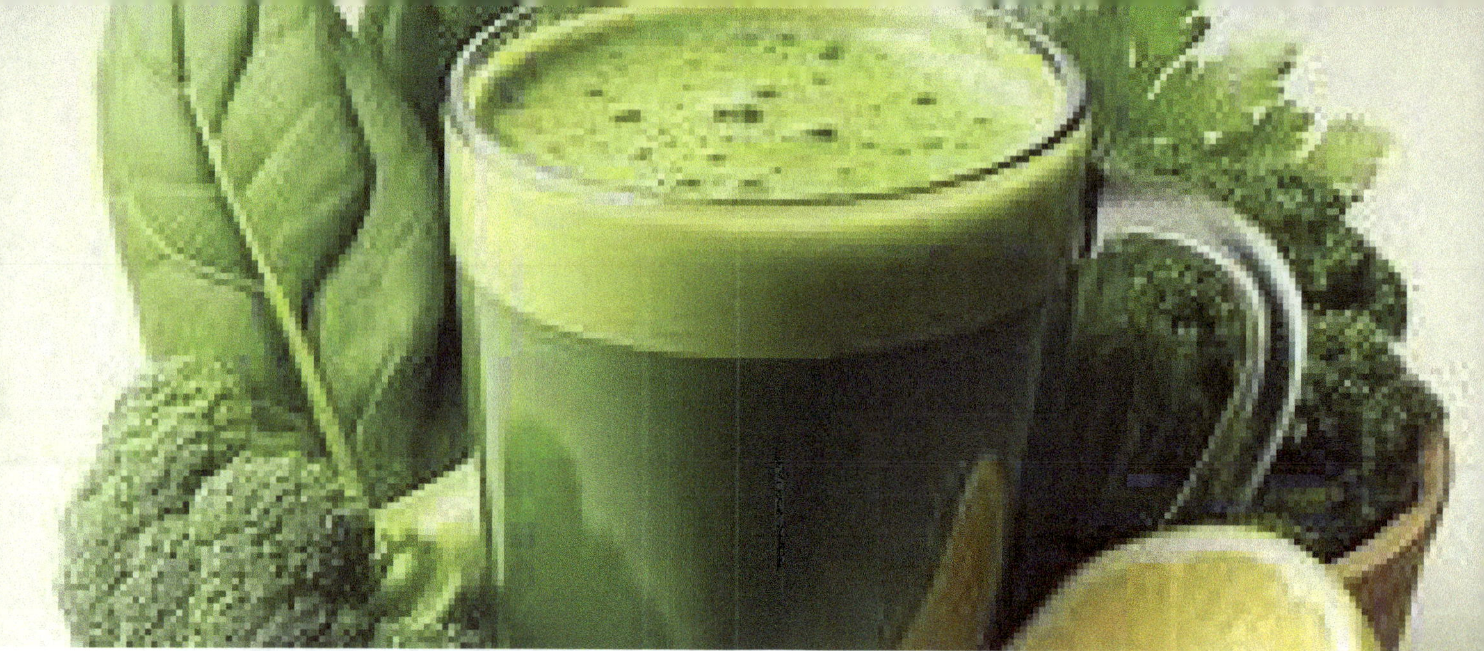

28. The Bone Builder Juice

Introduction:

This juice is designed to help strengthen bones and reduce the risk of osteoporosis. The ingredients in this juice are all good sources of calcium, magnesium, and vitamin K, which are essential for bone health.

Ingredients:

1 cup spinach

1/2 cup collard greens

1/4 cup parsley

1/4 cup lemon juice

Instructions:

Wash all of the ingredients well.

Cut the spinach and collard greens into small pieces.

Add all of the ingredients to a juicer and blend until smooth.

Serve immediately.

   Juicing for Cancer Recipes for Seniors

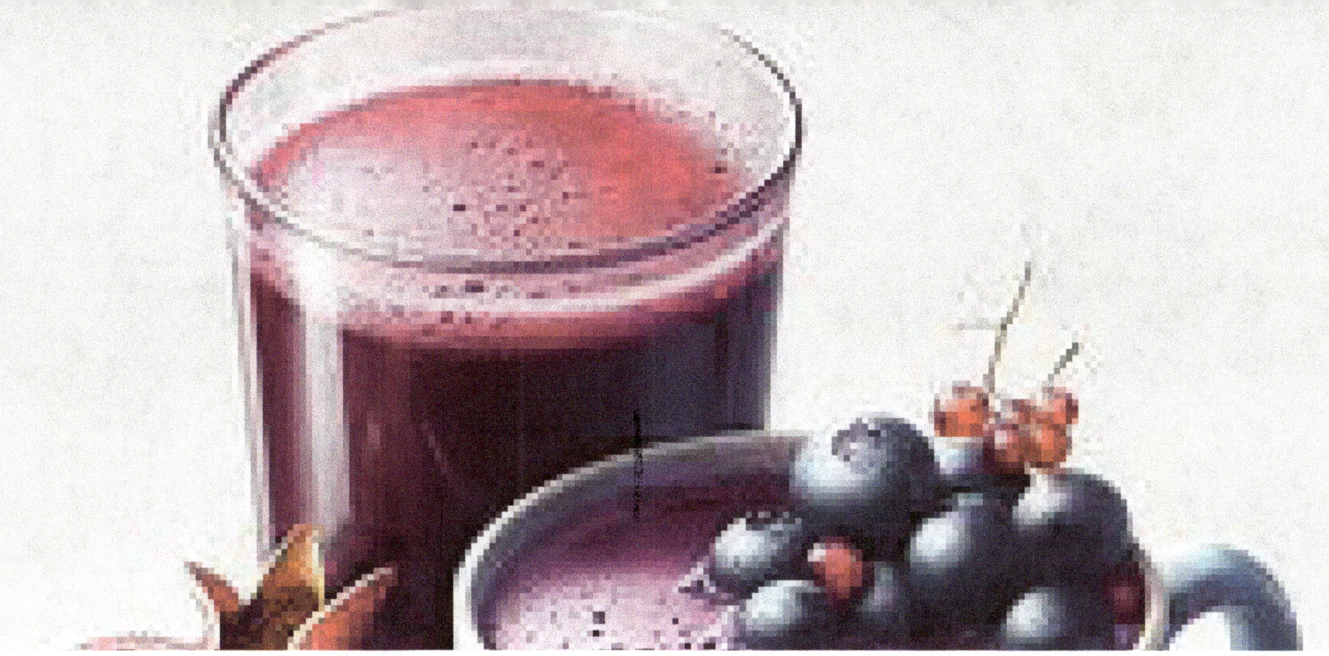

29. The Heart Protector Juice

Introduction:

This juice is designed to help protect the heart from disease. The ingredients in this juice, including pomegranate, blueberries, and turmeric, are all known to be beneficial for heart health.

Ingredients:

1/2 cup pomegranate seeds

1 cup blueberries

1/4 inch turmeric root, peeled and chopped

Instructions:

Wash all of the ingredients well.

Add all of the ingredients to a juicer and blend until smooth.

Serve immediately.

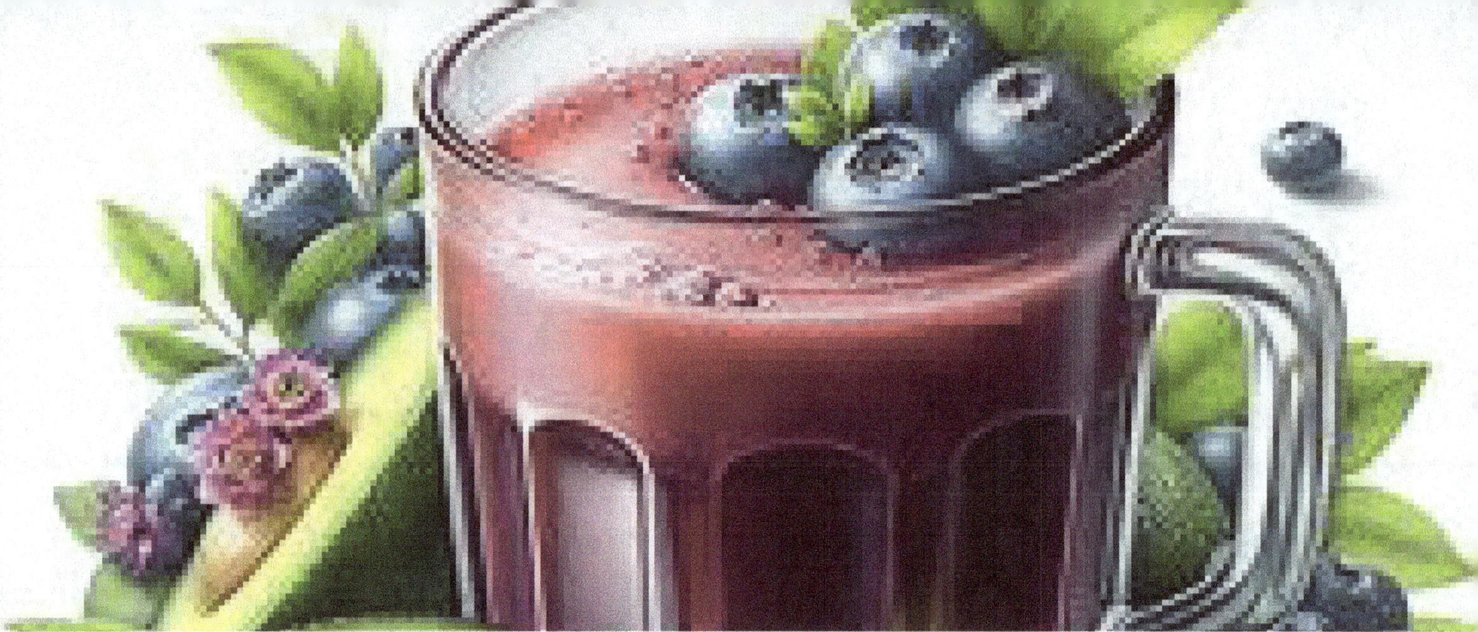

30. The Brain Booster Juice

Introduction:

This juice is made to boost brain function and improve memory. The ingredients in this juice, including blueberries, walnuts, and avocado, are all known to be beneficial for brain health.

Ingredients:

1 cup blueberries

1/4 cup walnuts

1/4 avocado

Instructions:

Wash all of the ingredients well.

Add all of the ingredients to a juicer and blend until smooth.

Serve immediately.

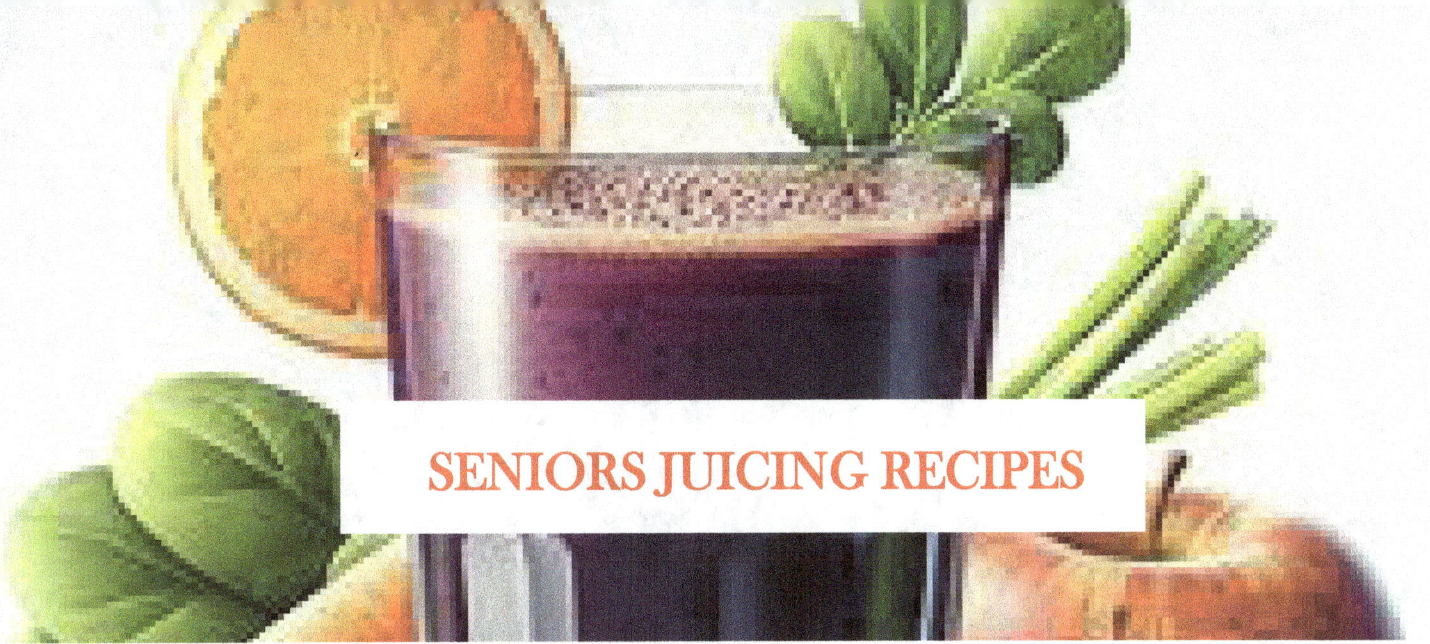

31. The Senior's Morning Boost

Introduction:

This refreshing juice is high in nutrients that can assist seniors' energy levels and cognitive function. It is also high in antioxidants, which can help protect the body from harm.

Ingredients:

1 carrot

1 apple

1/2 cup blueberries

1/2 cup spinach

1/2 cup water

Instructions:

Wash all of the ingredients well.

Cut the carrot and apple into small pieces.

Add all of the ingredients to a juicer and blend until smooth.

Serve immediately.

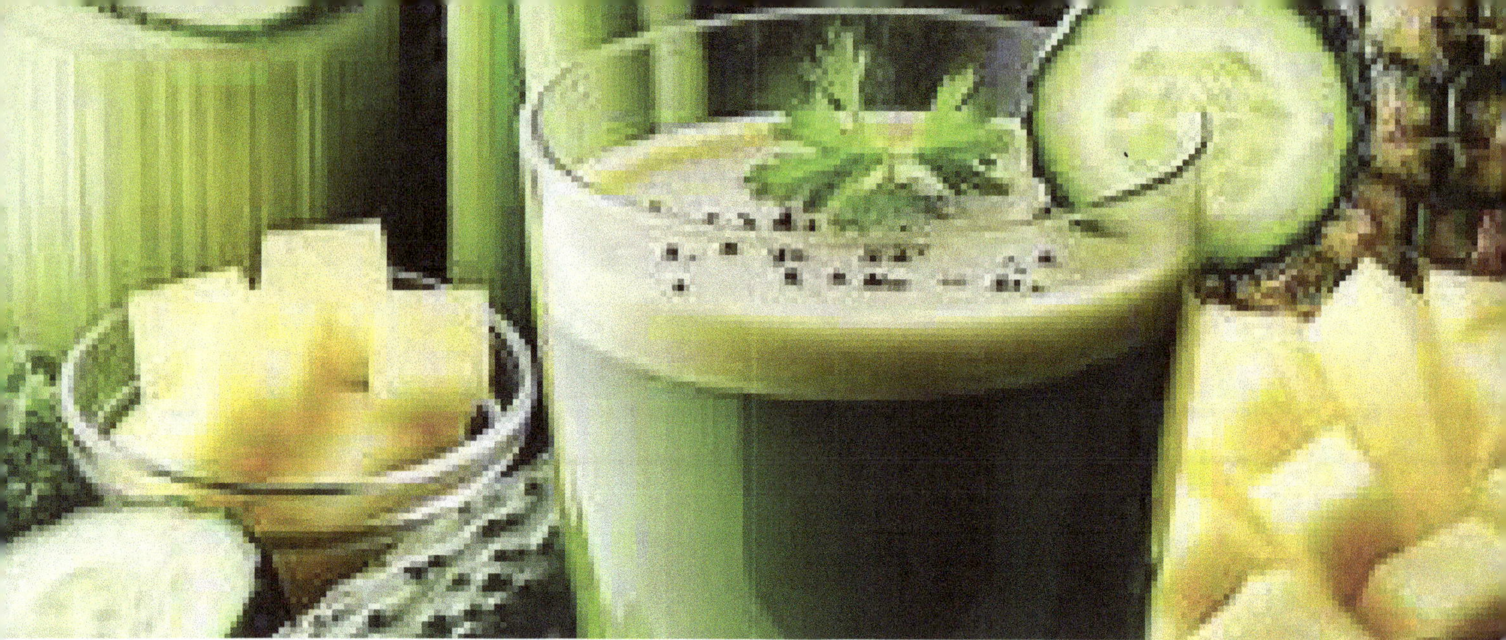

32. The Senior's Digestive

Introduction:

This juice is designed to help improve digestion and detoxify the body in seniors. It is a good source of fiber, vitamins, minerals, and antioxidants.

Ingredients:

1 cucumber

1 celery stalk

1/2 cup pineapple

1/2 cup kale

1/2 cup water

Instructions:

Wash all of the ingredients well.

Cut the beet into small pieces.

Add all of the ingredients to a juicer and blend until smooth.

Serve immediately.

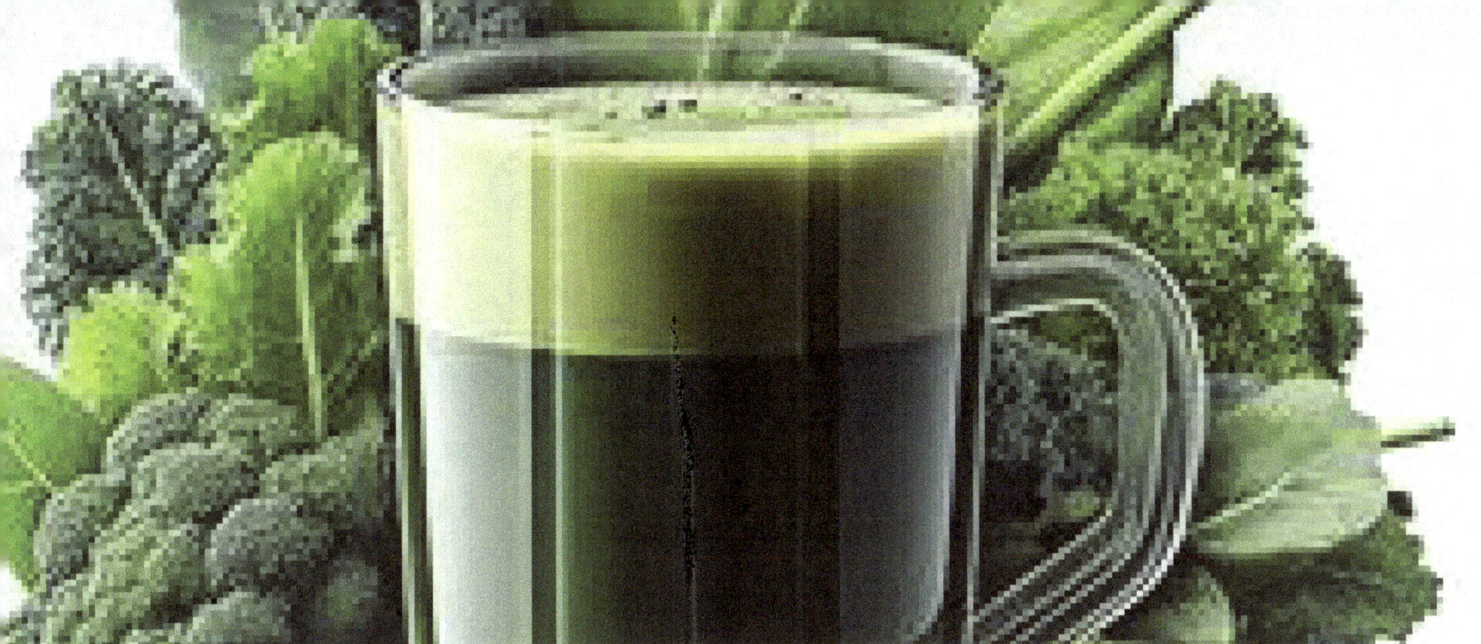

33. The Senior's Bone Builder

Introduction:

This juice is designed to assist in bone strengthening and lower the incidence of osteoporosis in seniors. It is high in magnesium, calcium, and vitamin K, all required for bone health.

Ingredients:

1 cup collard greens

1/2 cup spinach

1/2 cup kale

1/4 cup parsley

1/2 cup water

Instructions:

Wash all of the ingredients well.

Cut the cucumber, celery stalk, and pineapple into small pieces.

Add all of the ingredients to a juicer and blend until smooth.

Serve immediately.

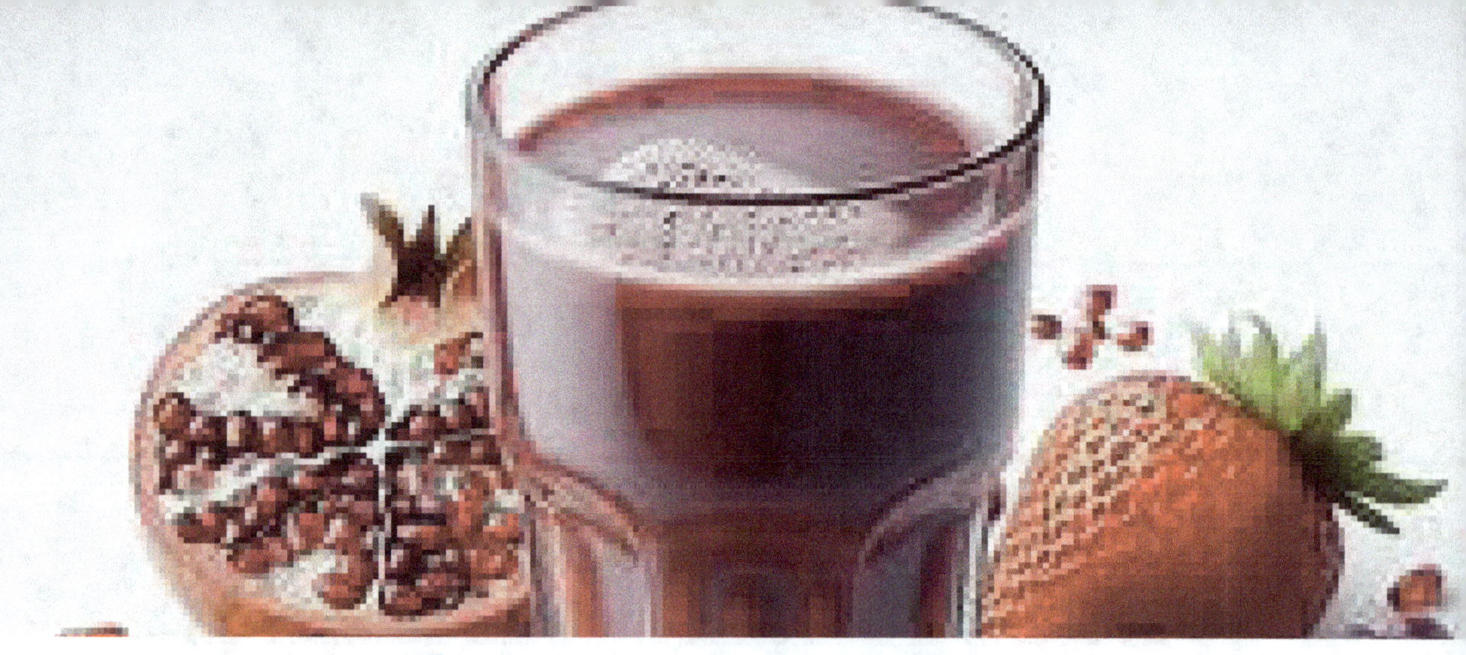

34. The Senior's Heart Protector

Introduction:

This juice is designed to help protect the heart from disease in seniors. It is high in vitamins, minerals, and antioxidants, which can aid in improving heart health.

Ingredients:

1 cup blueberries

1/2 cup strawberries

1/2 cup pomegranate seeds

1/2 cup water

Instructions:

Wash all of the ingredients well.

Cut the strawberries into small pieces.

Add all of the ingredients to a juicer and blend until smooth.

Serve immediately.

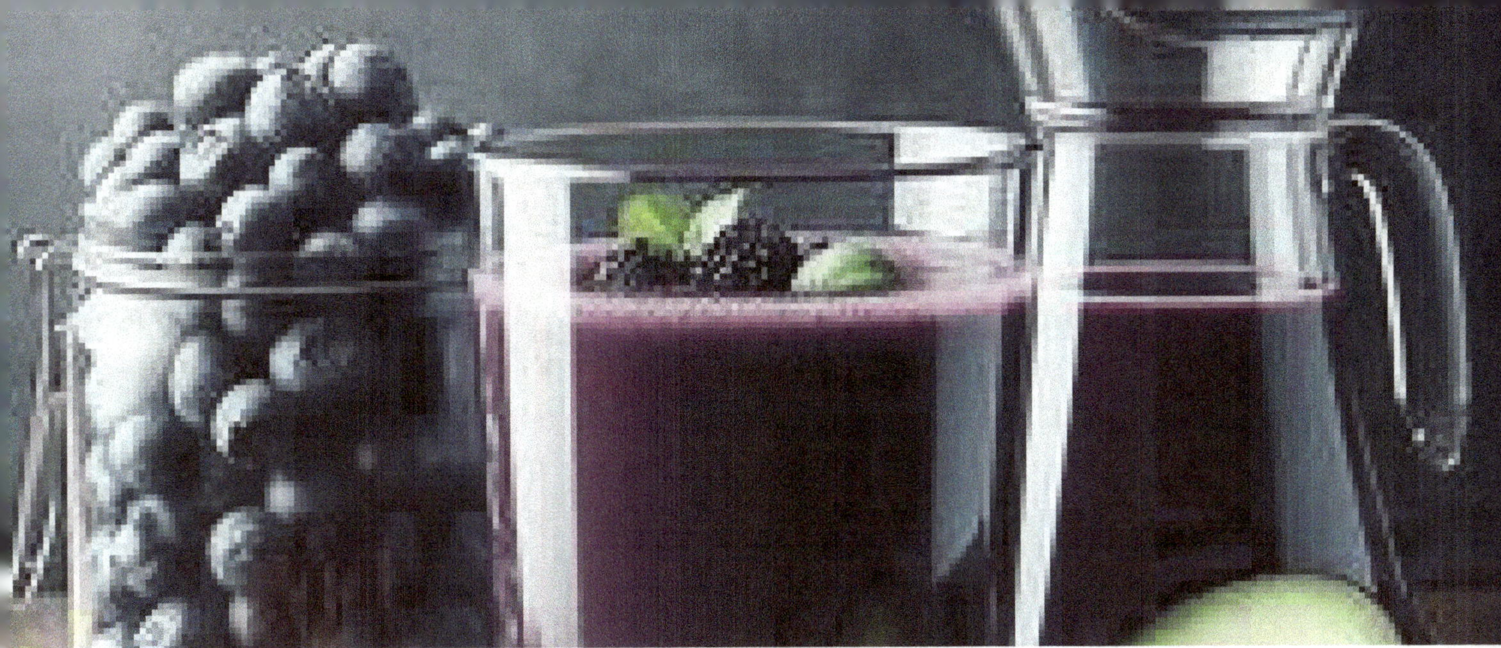

35. The Senior's Brain Booster

Introduction:

This juice is designed to boost brain function and improve memory in seniors. It is high in minerals, antioxidants, and vitamins, all of which can aid in protecting the brain from damage.

Ingredients:

1 cup blueberries

1/2 cup avocado

1/4 cup walnuts

1/2 cup water

Instructions:

Wash all of the ingredients well.

Cut the avocado into small pieces.

Add all of the ingredients to a juicer and blend until smooth.

Serve immediately.

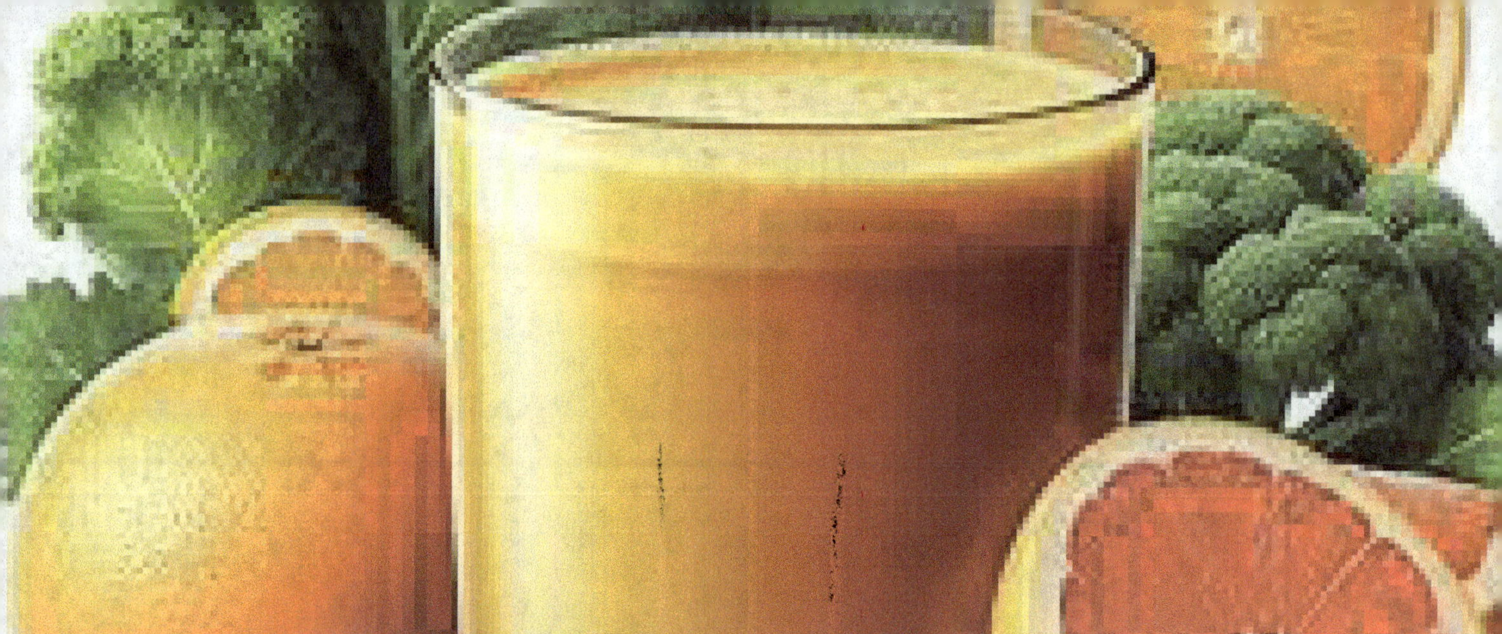

36. The Senior's Immune Booster

Introduction:

This juice is designed to boost the immune system and protect against infection in seniors. It is a good source of vitamin C, zinc, and antioxidants essential for immune function.

Ingredients:

1 orange

1 grapefruit

1/2 cup kale

1/4 cup ginger

1/4 cup water

Instructions:

Wash all of the ingredients well.

Cut the orange, grapefruit, and kale into small pieces.

Add all of the ingredients to a juicer and blend until smooth.

Serve immediately.

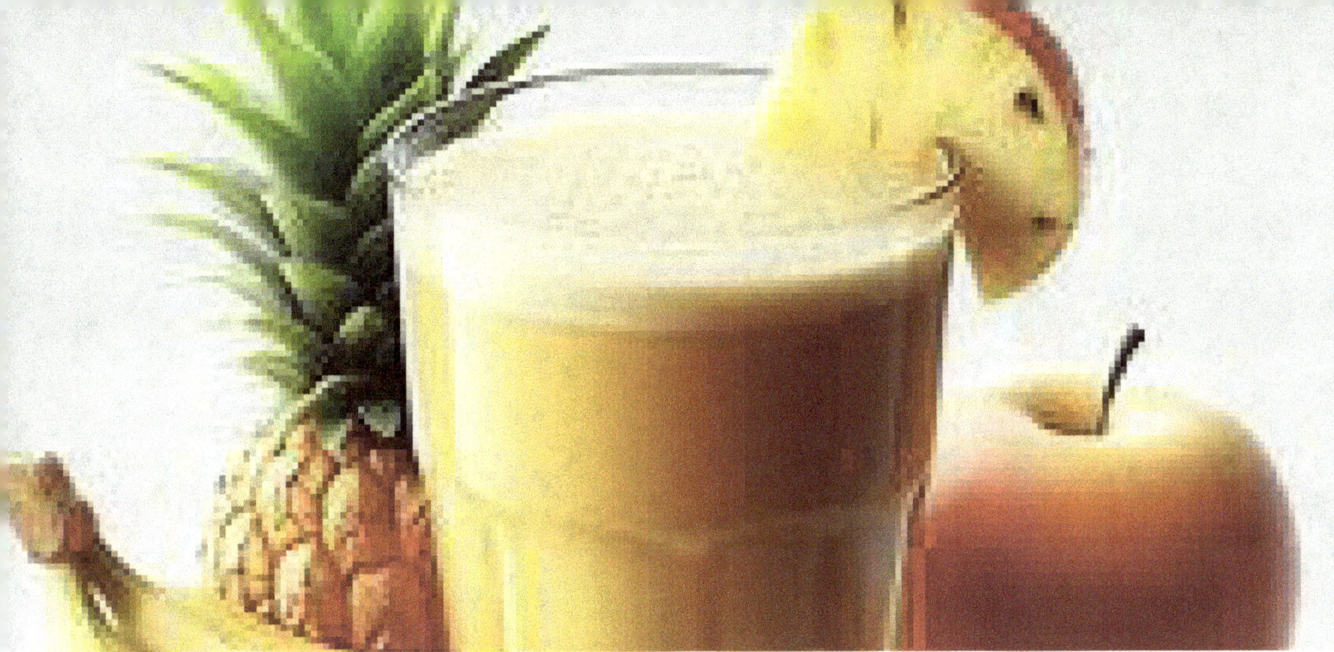

37. The Senior's Energy Booster

Introduction:

This juice is designed to boost energy levels and reduce fatigue in seniors. It is a good source of natural sugars, electrolytes, and vitamins, which can help to improve energy production.

Ingredients:

1 banana

1 apple

1/2 cup pineapple

1/2 cup coconut water

Instructions:

Wash all of the ingredients well.

Cut the banana, apple, and pineapple into small pieces.

Add all of the ingredients to a juicer and blend until smooth.

Serve immediately.

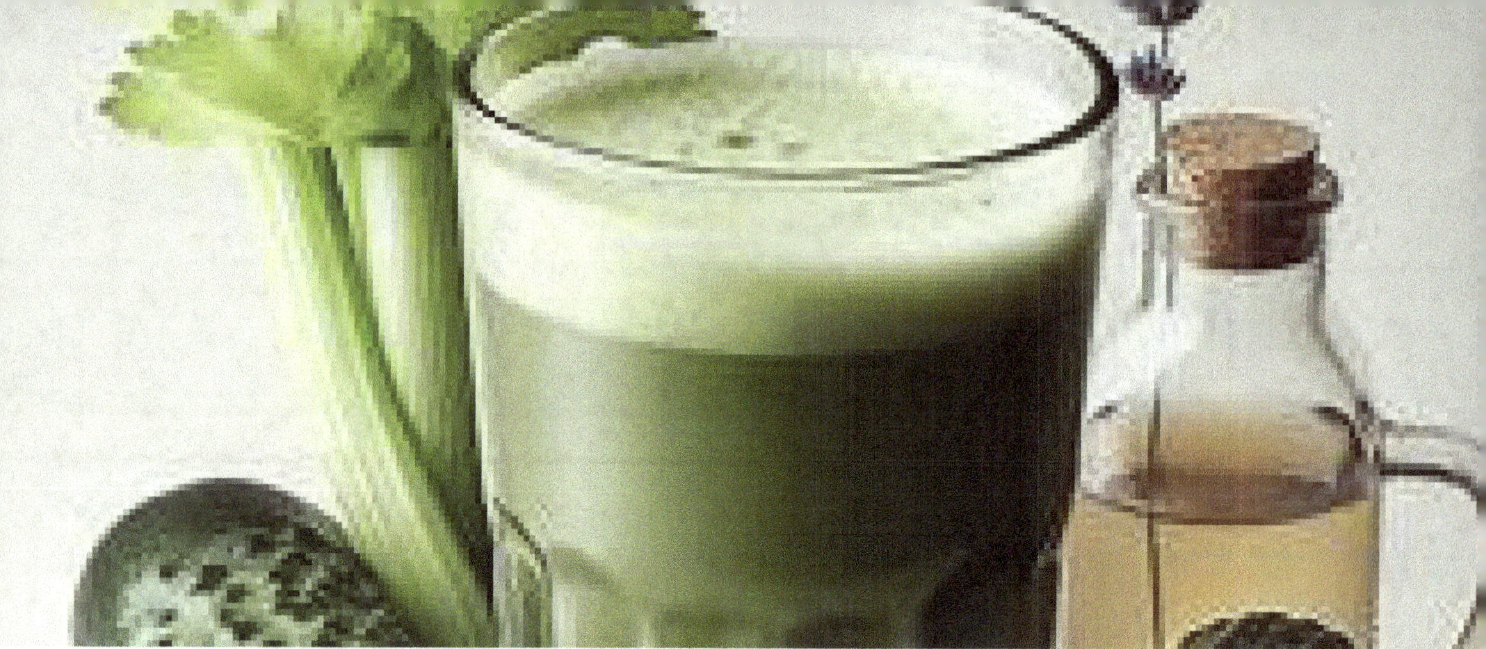

38. The Senior's Sleep Promoter

Introduction:

This juice is designed to help improve sleep quality in seniors. It contains components that have been found to support relaxation and stress reduction, such as chamomile and lavender.

Ingredients:

1 cucumber

1/2 cup celery

1/4 cup chamomile tea

1/4 cup lavender tea

Instructions:

Wash all of the ingredients well.

Cut the cucumber and celery into small pieces.

Combine the cucumber, celery, chamomile, and lavender tea in a blender and mix until smooth.

Serve immediately.

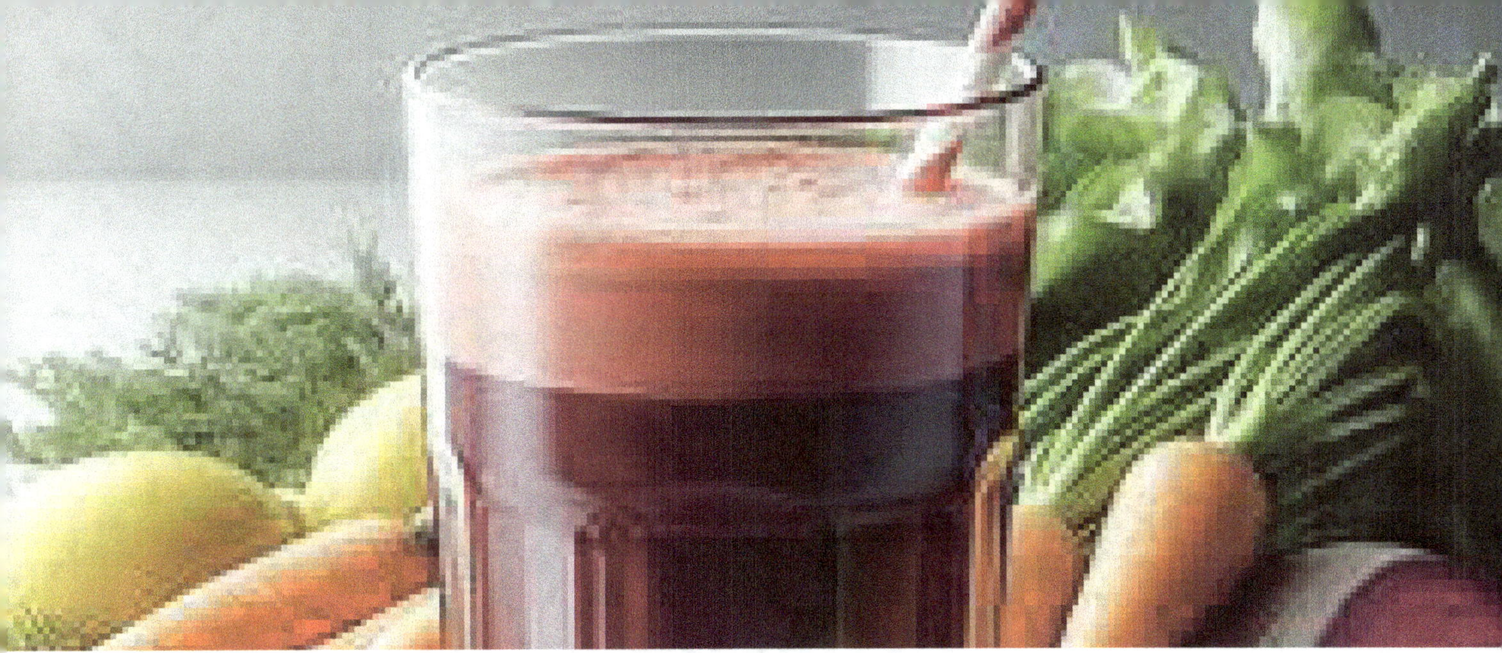

39. The Senior's Detoxifier

Introduction:

This juice is designed to help detoxify the body and remove harmful toxins in seniors. It contains ingredients that support liver function, such as beets, carrots, and turmeric.

Ingredients:

1 beet

2 carrots

1/2 inch turmeric root, peeled and chopped

1/4 cup lemon juice

Instructions:

Wash all of the ingredients well.

Cut the beet into small pieces.

Add all of the ingredients to a juicer and blend until smooth.

Serve immediately.

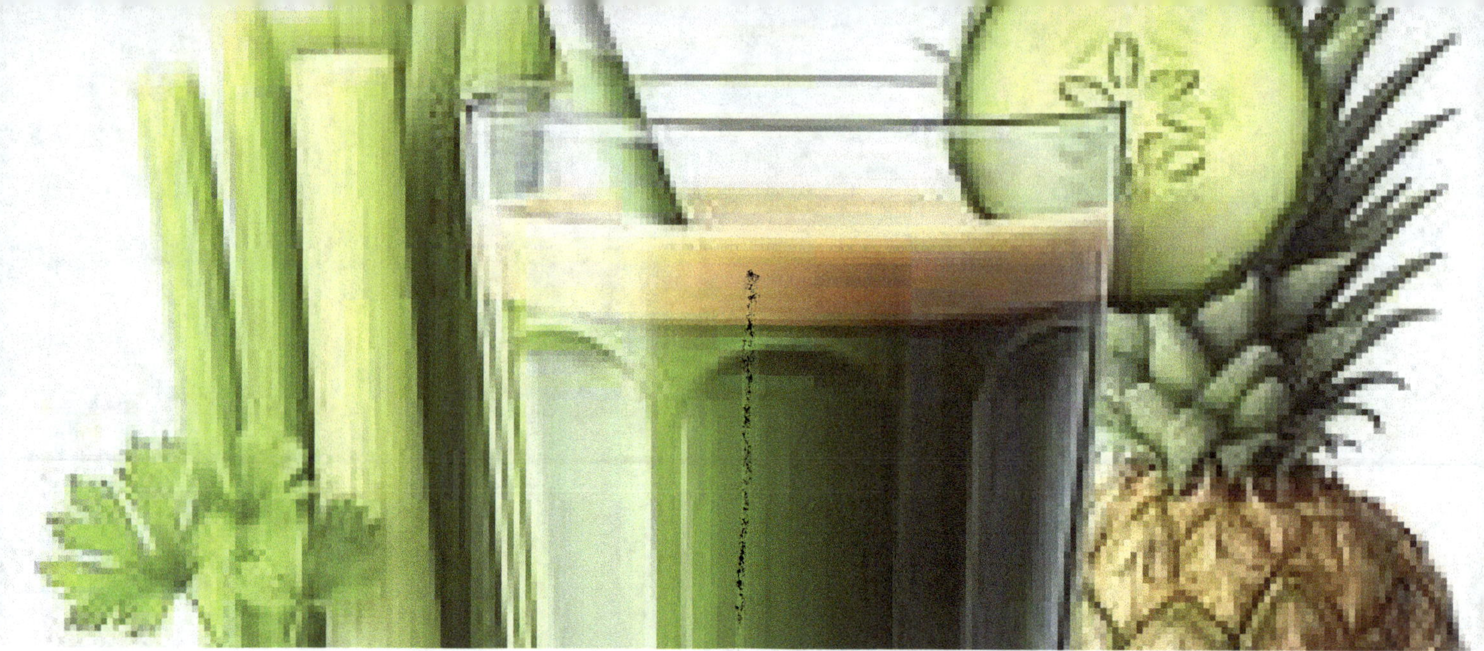

40. The Senior's Anti-Inflammatory

Introduction:

This juice is designed to reduce inflammation and improve joint function in seniors. It contains ingredients that are known to have anti-inflammatory properties, such as ginger, turmeric, and pineapple.

Ingredients:

1/2 cucumber

1/2 cup celery

1/4 cup pineapple

1/4 inch turmeric root, peeled and chopped

1/4 teaspoon ginger, peeled and grated

Instructions:

Wash all of the ingredients well.

Cut the cucumber, celery, and pineapple into small pieces.

Add all of the ingredients to a juicer and blend until smooth.

Serve immediately.

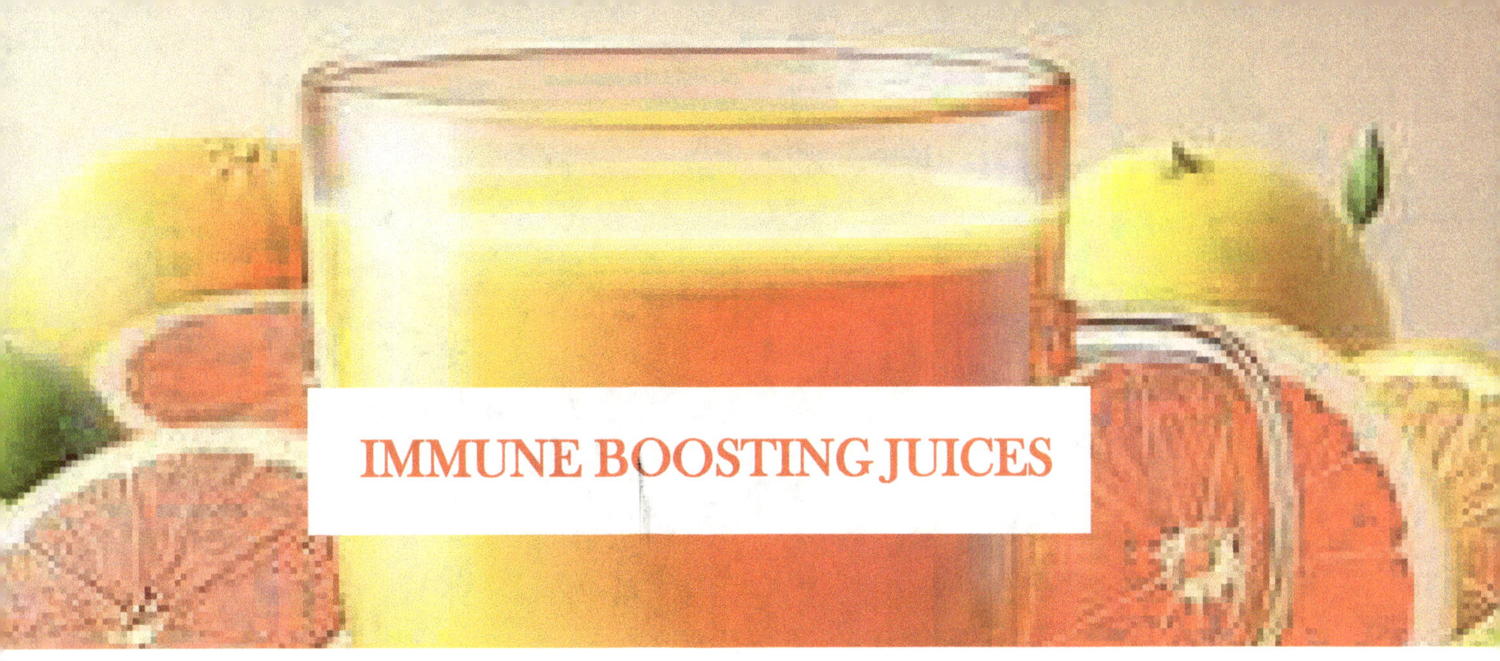

41. The Immune-Boosting Citrus

Introduction:

This juice is high in vitamin C and other valuable antioxidants that can enhance the immune system and fight against illness. The citrus fruits in this juice are also a good source of electrolytes, which can help to keep you hydrated and energized.

Ingredients:

1 orange

1 grapefruit

1 lemon

1/2 cup lime juice

Instructions:

Wash all of the ingredients well.

Cut the orange, grapefruit, and lemon into small pieces.

Add all of the ingredients to a juicer and blend until smooth.

Serve immediately.

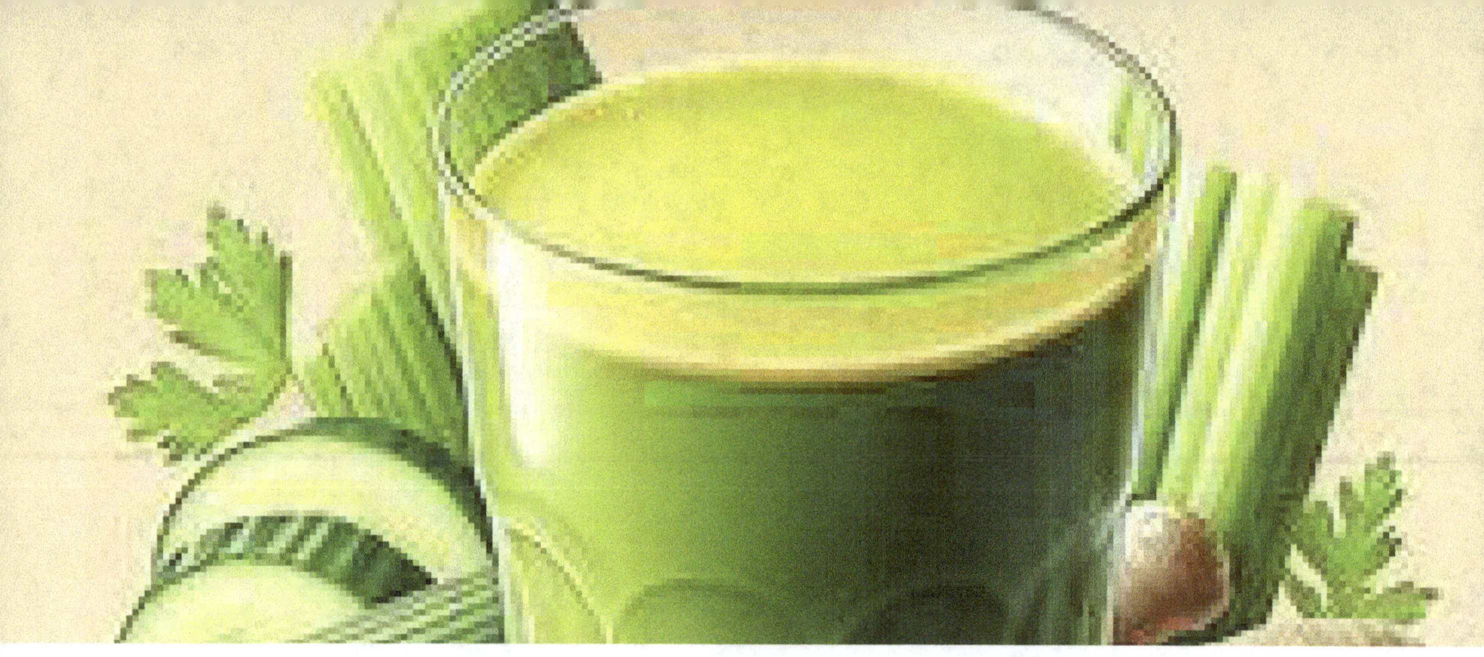

42. The Ginger-Turmeric Kick

Introduction:

This juice is rich in ginger and turmeric, two spices with powerful anti-inflammatory and immune-boosting properties. The ginger in this juice can also help to soothe the stomach and reduce nausea.

Ingredients:

1 cucumber

1/2 cup celery

1/4 inch peeled and sliced ginger root

1/4 inch turmeric root, peeled and chopped

Instructions:

Wash all of the ingredients well.

Cut the cucumber and celery into small pieces.

Add all of the ingredients to a juicer and blend until smooth.

Serve immediately.

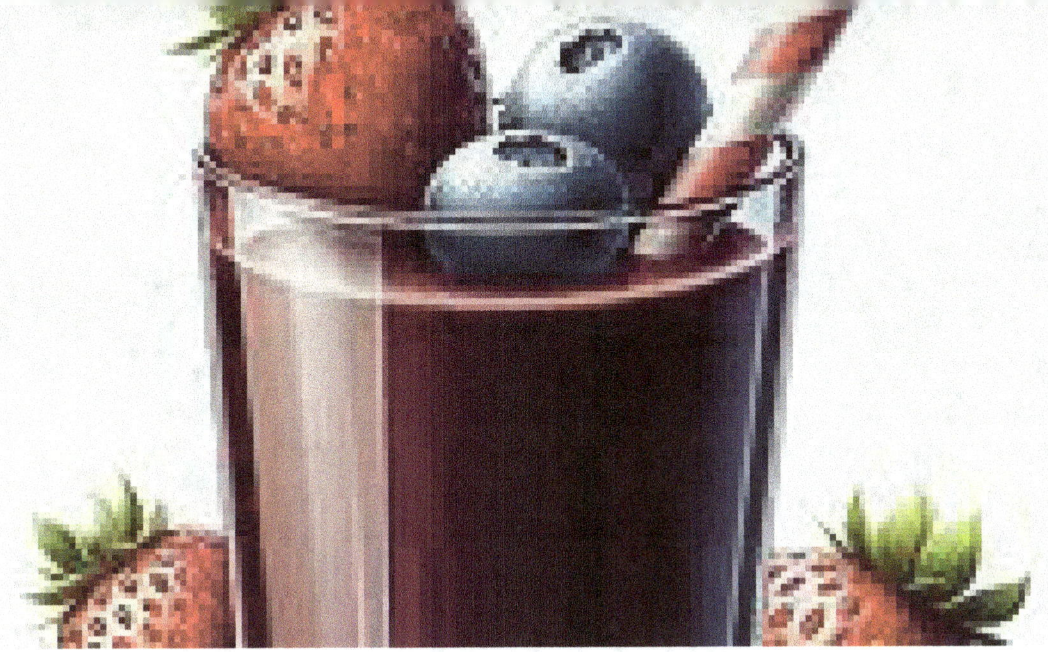

43. The Berry Blast Juice

Introduction:

This juice contains berries, a great source of antioxidants and vitamins. The berries contained in this juice can help improve the immune system, decrease inflammation, and protect against heart disease.

Ingredients:

1 cup blueberries

1 cup strawberries

1/2 cup raspberries

1/2 cup blackberries

Instructions:

Wash all of the ingredients well.

Cut the beet into small pieces.

Add all of the ingredients to a juicer and blend until smooth.

Serve immediately.

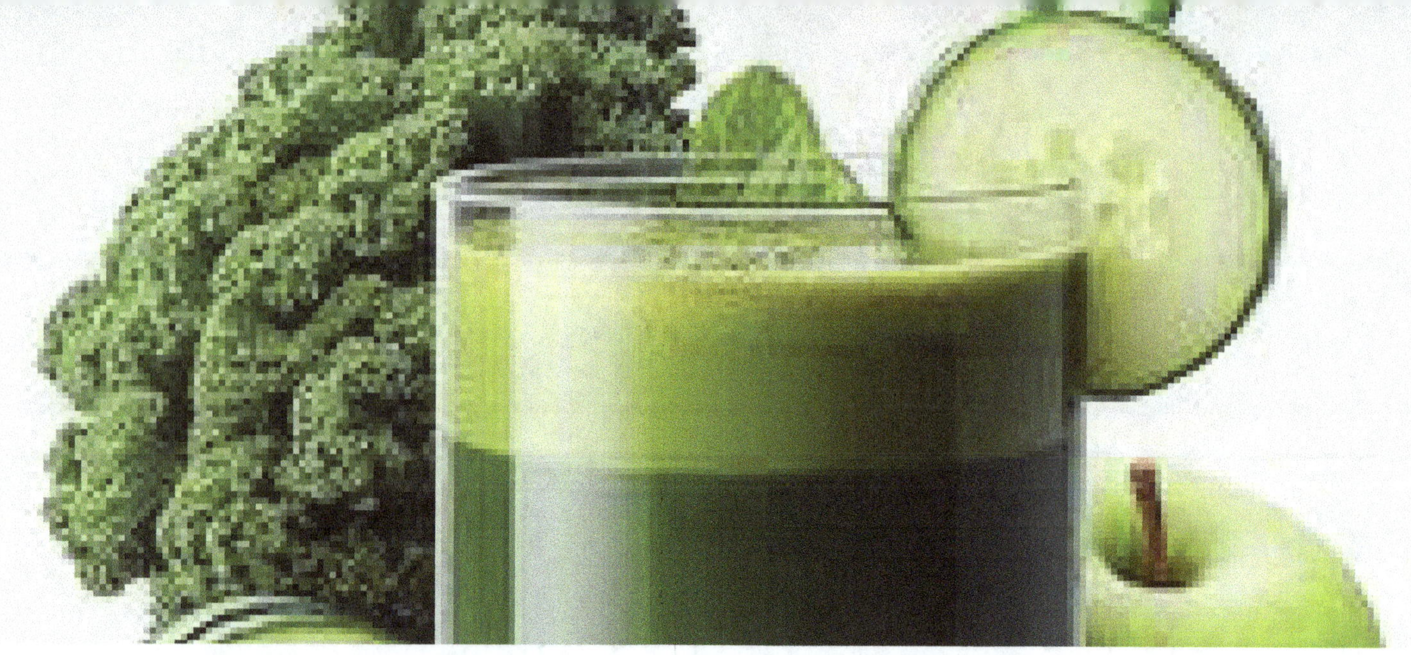

44. The Green Machine

Introduction:

This juice is packed with leafy green vegetables rich in minerals and antioxidants. The leafy greens in this juice enhance the immune system, minimize inflammation, and promote digestion.

Ingredients:

1 cup kale

1 cup spinach

1/2 cucumber

1/2 green apple

Instructions:

Wash all of the ingredients well.

Cut the cucumber and apple into small pieces.

Add all of the ingredients to a juicer and blend until smooth.

Serve immediately.

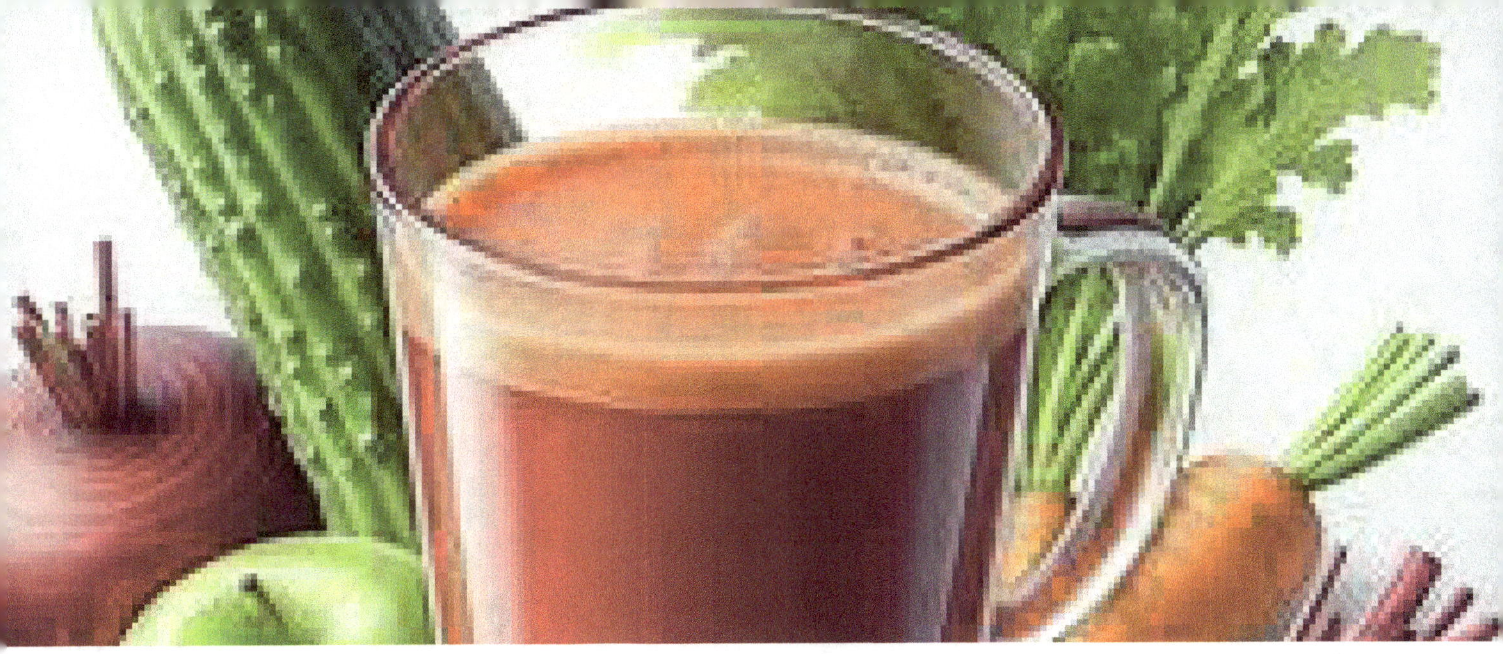

45. The Carrot-Beet Boost

Introduction:

This juice is packed with carrots and beets, which are excellent sources of nutrients such as vitamins, minerals, and antioxidants. The carrots and beets in this juice may promote the immune system, improve eyesight, and lower the risk of heart disease.

Ingredients:

1 cup carrots

1 beet

1/2 cucumber

1/2 green apple

Instructions:

Wash all of the ingredients well.

Cut the carrots, beet, cucumber, and apple into small pieces.

Add all of the ingredients to a juicer and blend until smooth.

Serve immediately.

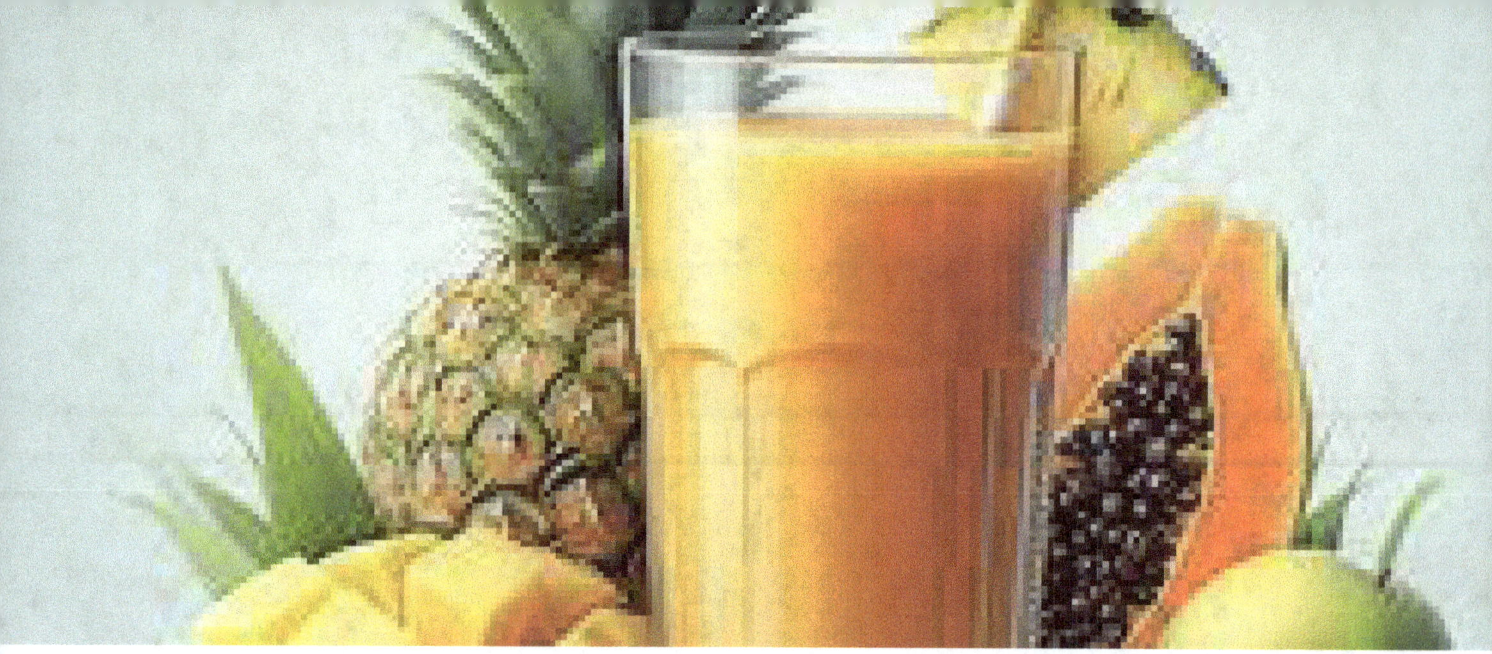

46. The Tropical Immunity Boost

Introduction:

This juice is packed with tropical fruits and contains vitamins, minerals, and antioxidants. The tropical fruits in this juice enhance the immune system, minimize inflammation, and improve digestion.

Ingredients:

1 cup pineapple

1 cup mango

1/2 cup papaya

1/2 cup coconut water

Instructions:

Wash all of the ingredients well.

Cut the pineapple, mango, and papaya into small pieces.

Add all of the ingredients to a juicer and blend until smooth.

Serve immediately.

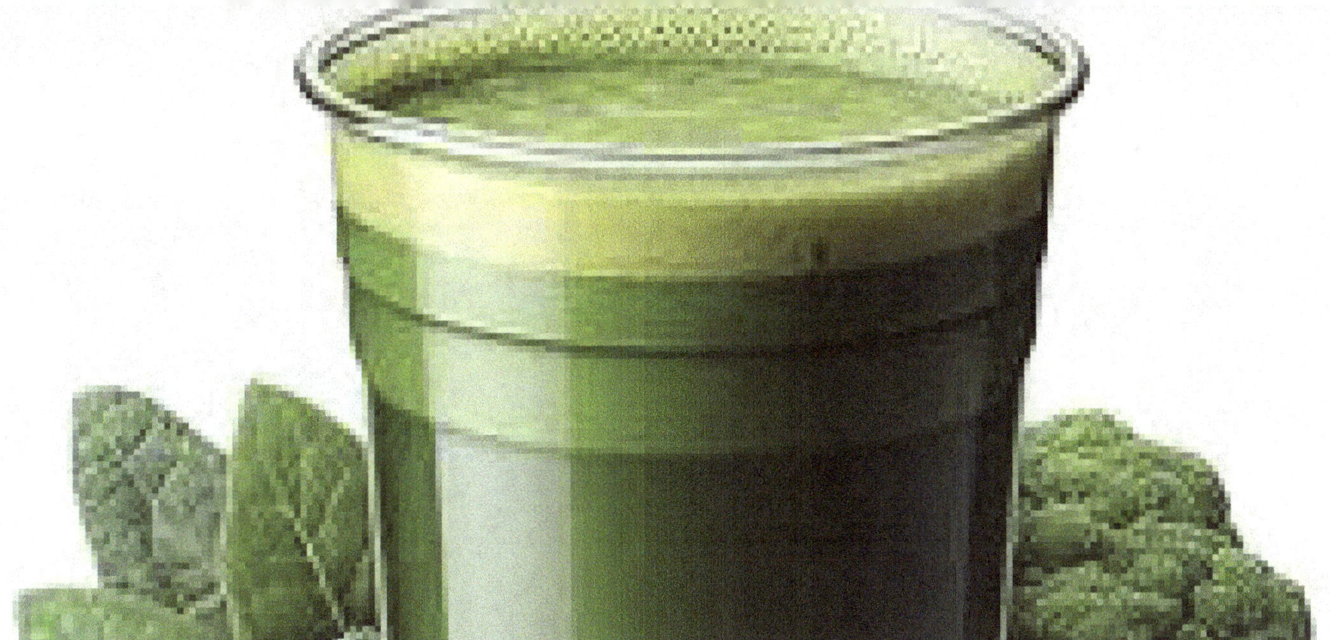

47. The Spicy Greens Cleanse

Introduction:

This juice is packed with leafy green vegetables and spices, which can help to cleanse the body and boost the immune system. The leafy greens in this juice are rich in mineral content, vitamins, and antioxidants, and the spices have anti-inflammatory and antimicrobial properties.

Ingredients:

1 cup kale

1 cup spinach

1/2 cucumber

1/4 inch peeled and sliced ginger root

1/4 teaspoon cayenne pepper

Instructions:

Wash all of the ingredients well.

Cut the cucumber into small pieces.

Add all of the ingredients to a juicer and blend until smooth.

Serve immediately.

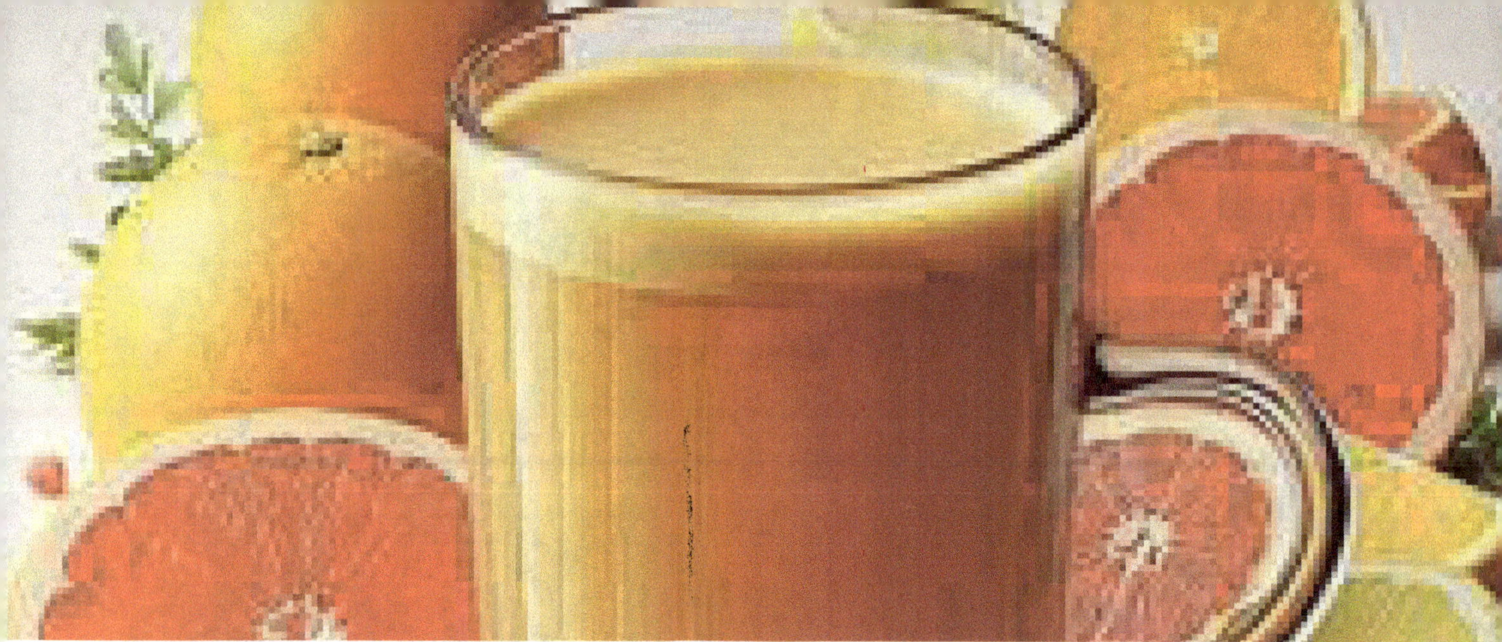

48. The Citrus-Ginger Detox

Introduction:

This juice is packed with citrus fruits and ginger, which can help to detoxify the body and boost the immune system. The citrus fruits in this juice are a good source of vitamin C, while the ginger has anti-inflammatory and antimicrobial properties.

Ingredients:

1 orange

1 grapefruit

1 lemon

1/2 inch peeled and chopped ginger root

Instructions:

Wash all of the ingredients well.

Cut the orange, grapefruit, and lemon into small pieces.

Add all of the ingredients to a juicer and blend until smooth.

Serve immediately.

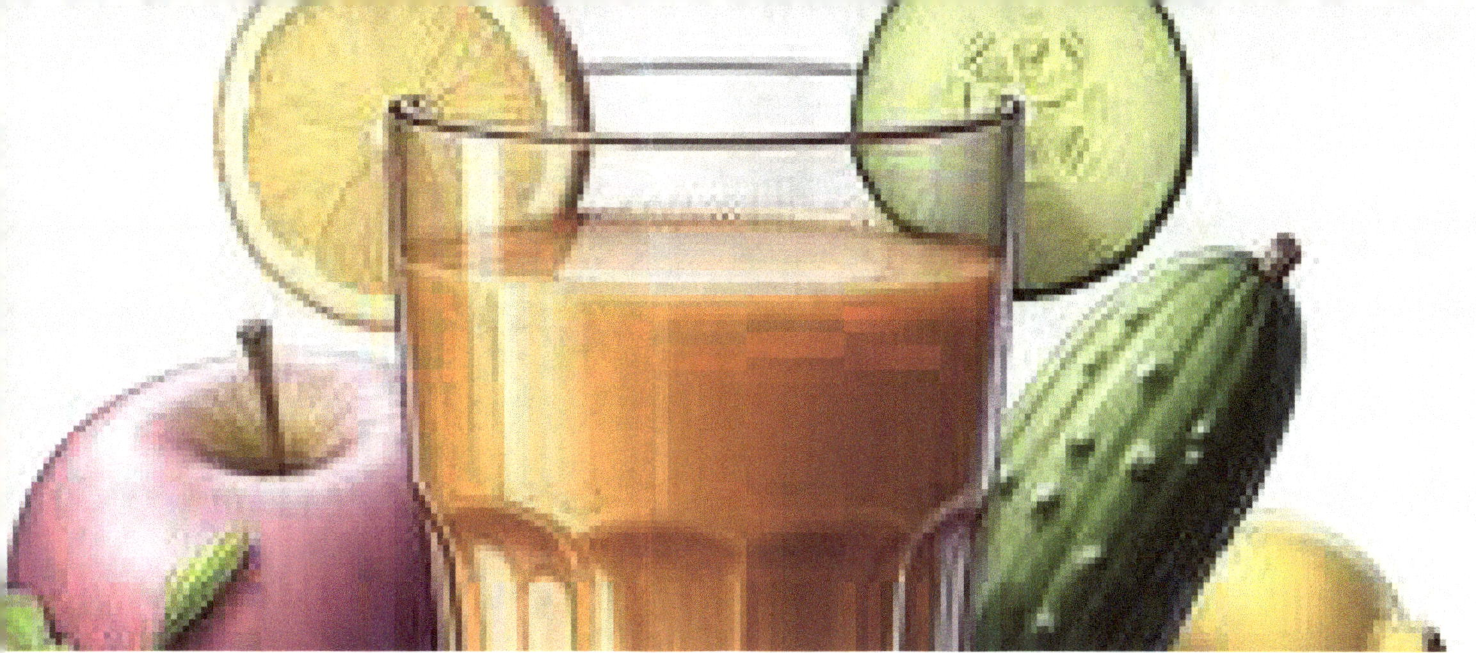

49. The Sweet Potato Boost

Introduction:

This juice is packed with sweet potato, a good source of vitamins, minerals, and antioxidants. Sweet potato is also a good source of carbohydrates, which can provide energy.

Ingredients:

1 cup sweet potato, peeled and cubed

1 apple

1/2 cucumber

1/2 lemon, peeled and juiced

Instructions:

Wash all of the ingredients well.

Cut the sweet potato, apple, and cucumber into small pieces.

Add all of the ingredients to a juicer and blend until smooth.

Serve immediately.

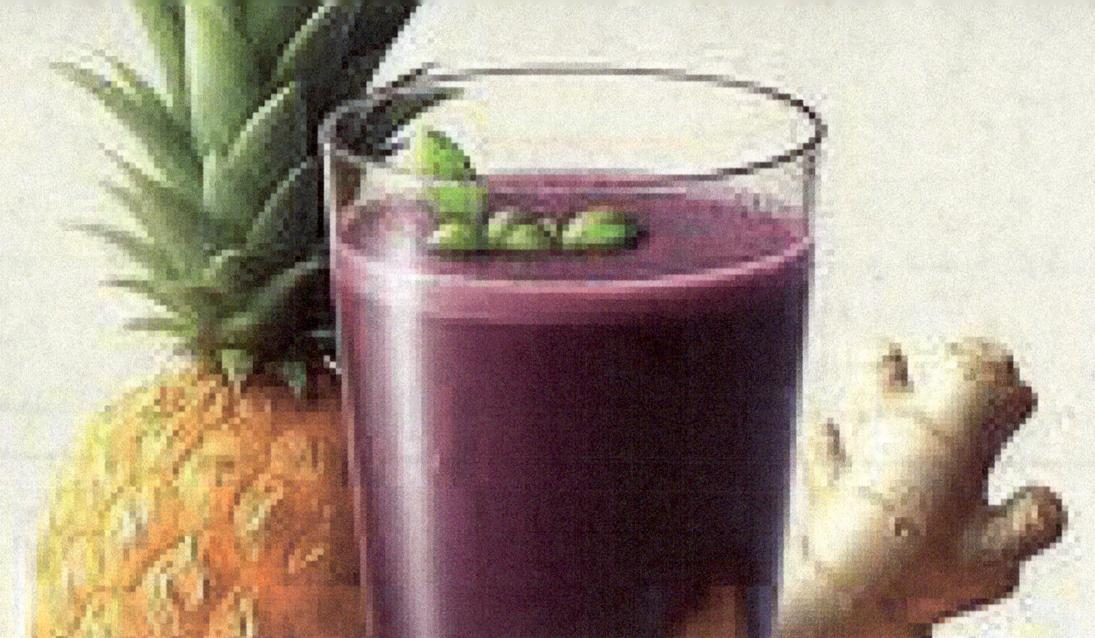

50. The Anti-Inflammatory Juice

Introduction:

This juice is packed with fruits and vegetables that have anti-inflammatory properties. The ingredients contained in this juice can help reduce general inflammation in the body, which can help with various illnesses such as arthritis, respiratory conditions, and cardiovascular disease.

Ingredients:

1 cup blueberries

1/2 cup pineapple

1/4 cup turmeric root, peeled and chopped

1/4 cup peeled and chopped ginger root

Instructions:

Wash all of the ingredients well.

Cut the pineapple and turmeric root into small pieces.

Add all of the ingredients to a juicer and blend until smooth.

Serve immediately.

    Juicing for Cancer Recipes for Seniors

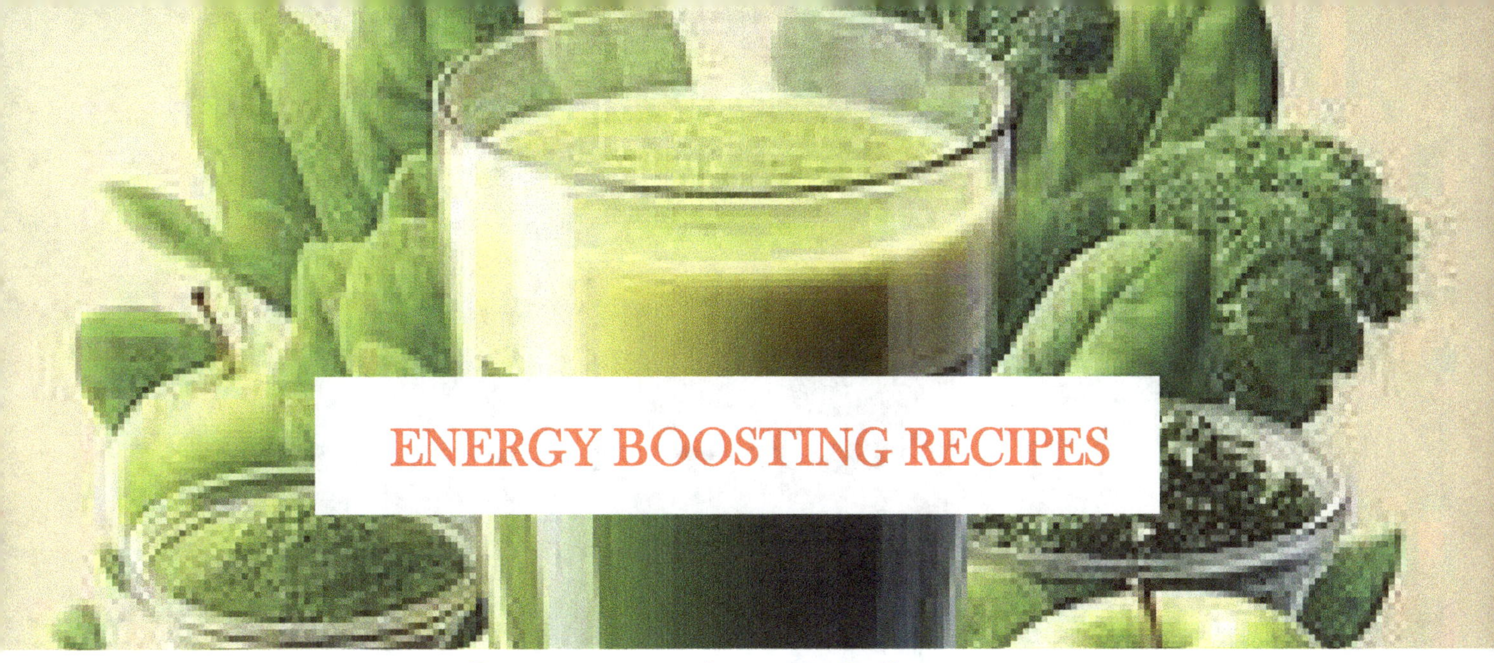

51. The Morning Kickstart

Introduction:

This juice is packed with ingredients that help you get going in the morning by increasing your energy levels. The apple and banana provide natural sugars and carbohydrates for energy, while the spinach and kale are high in vitamins and minerals necessary for cellular function.

Ingredients:

1 apple

1 banana

1 cup spinach

1/2 cup kale

1/2 cup water

Instructions:

Wash all of the ingredients well.

Cut the apple and banana into small pieces.

Add all of the ingredients to a juicer and blend until smooth.

Serve immediately.

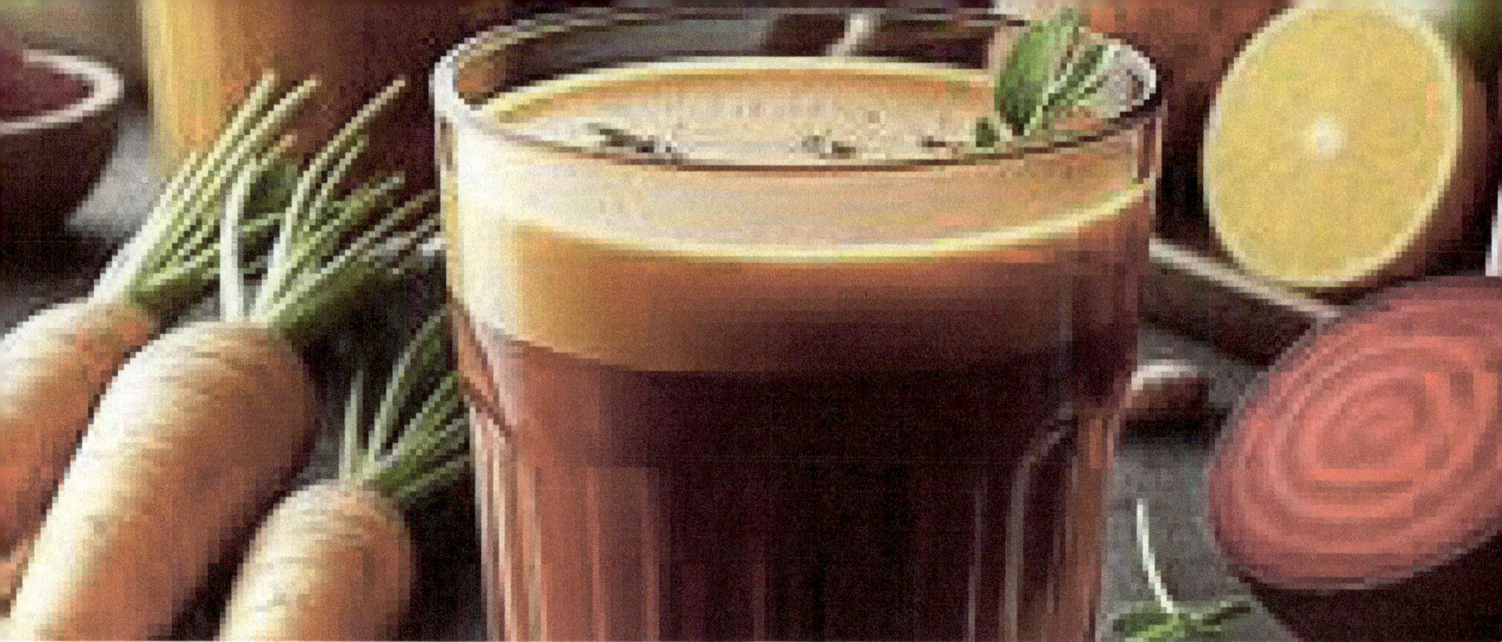

52. The Midday Boost

Introduction:

This juice is perfect for a midday energy pick-me-up. The carrots and beets are packed with essential vitamins and minerals for energy production, while ginger and turmeric's anti-inflammatory and antioxidant effects are widely recognized.

Ingredients:

1 cup carrots

1 beet

1/2 inch peeled and chopped ginger root

1/4 inch turmeric root, peeled and chopped

1/2 cup water

Instructions:

Wash all of the ingredients well.

Cut the carrots and beets into small pieces.

Add all of the ingredients to a juicer and blend until smooth.

Serve immediately.

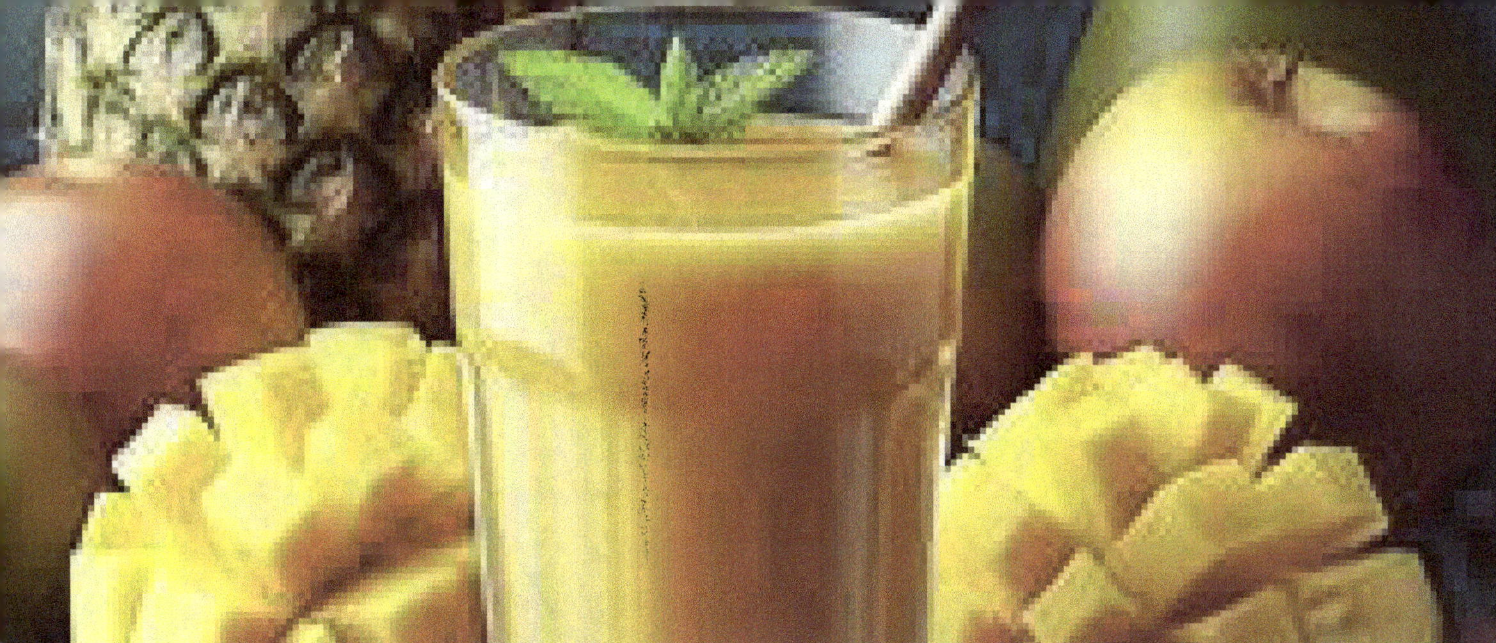

53. The Pre-Workout Fuel

Introduction:

Recipe #3: This juice is perfect for drinking before a workout. The pineapple and mango provide natural sugars and carbohydrates for energy, while the coconut water is a good source of electrolytes to keep you hydrated.

Ingredients:

1 cup pineapple

1 cup mango

1/2 cup coconut water

Instructions:

Wash all of the ingredients well.

Cut the pineapple and mango into small pieces.

Add all of the ingredients to a juicer and blend until smooth.

Serve immediately.

Juicing for Cancer Recipes for Seniors

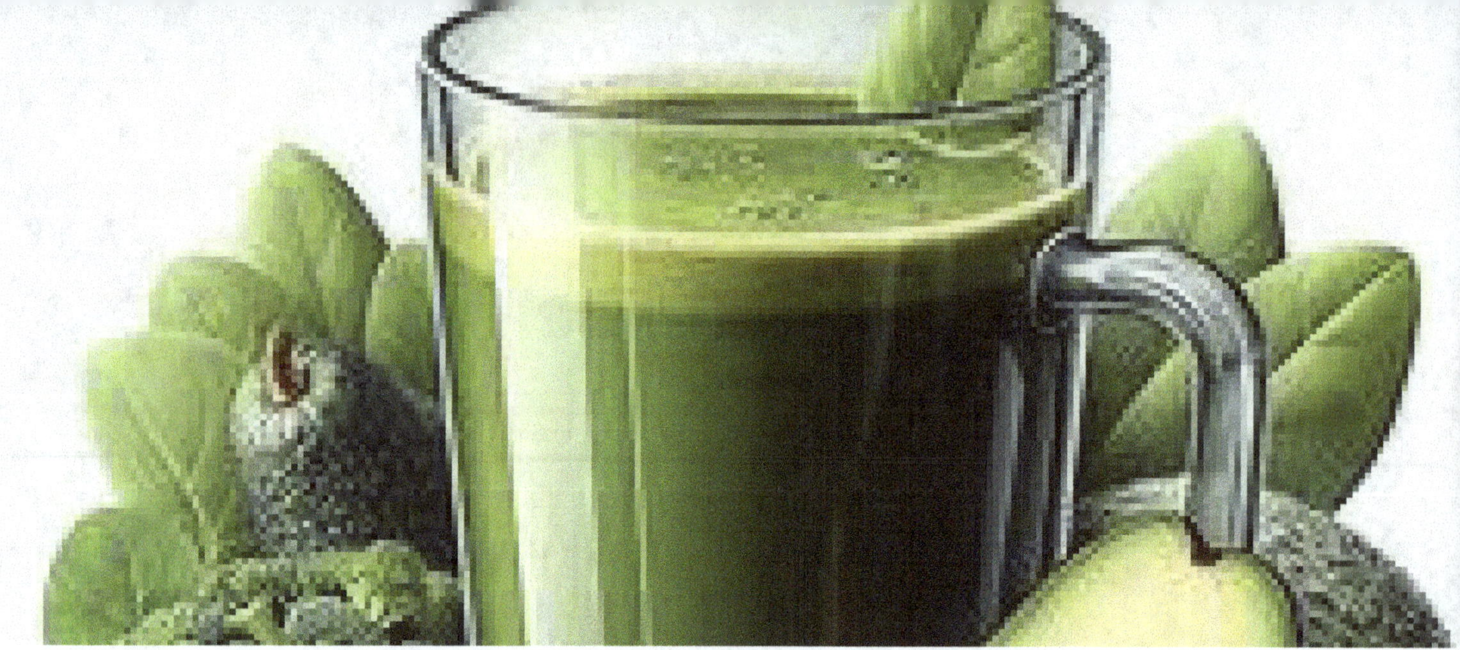

54. The All-Day Energy Booster

Introduction:

This juice is a great way to maintain energy levels throughout the day. The avocado and walnuts provide healthy fats and protein, while the spinach and kale contain vitamins and minerals.

Ingredients:

1/2 avocado

1/4 cup walnuts

1 cup spinach

1/2 cup kale

1/2 cup water

Instructions:

Wash all of the ingredients well.

Cut the avocado into small pieces.

Add all of the ingredients to a juicer and blend until smooth.

Serve immediately.

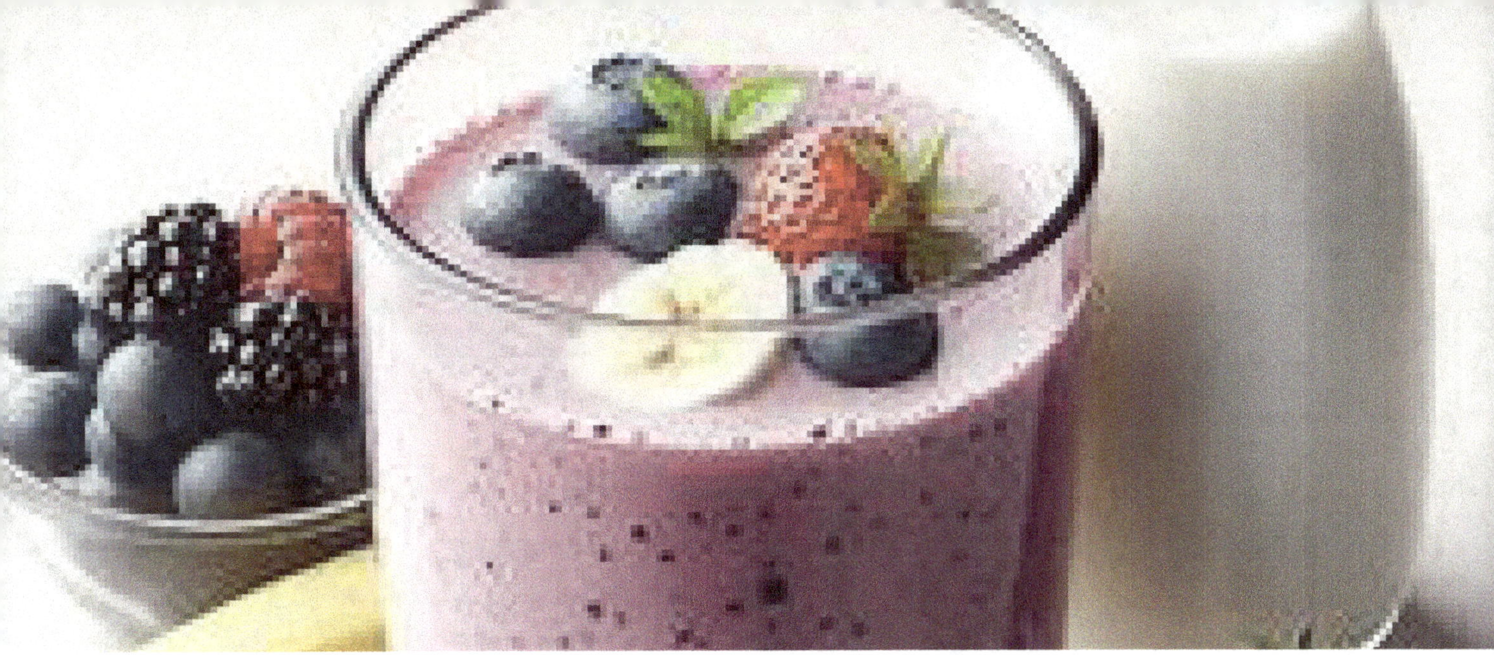

55. The Post-Workout Recovery

Introduction:

This juice is perfect for drinking after a workout. The berries and banana are packed with vitamins and minerals essential for muscle recovery, while the almond milk provides protein and healthy fats.

Ingredients:

1 cup berries

1 banana

1/2 cup almond milk

Instructions:

Wash all of the ingredients well.

Cut the banana into small pieces.

Add all of the ingredients to a juicer and blend until smooth.

Serve immediately.

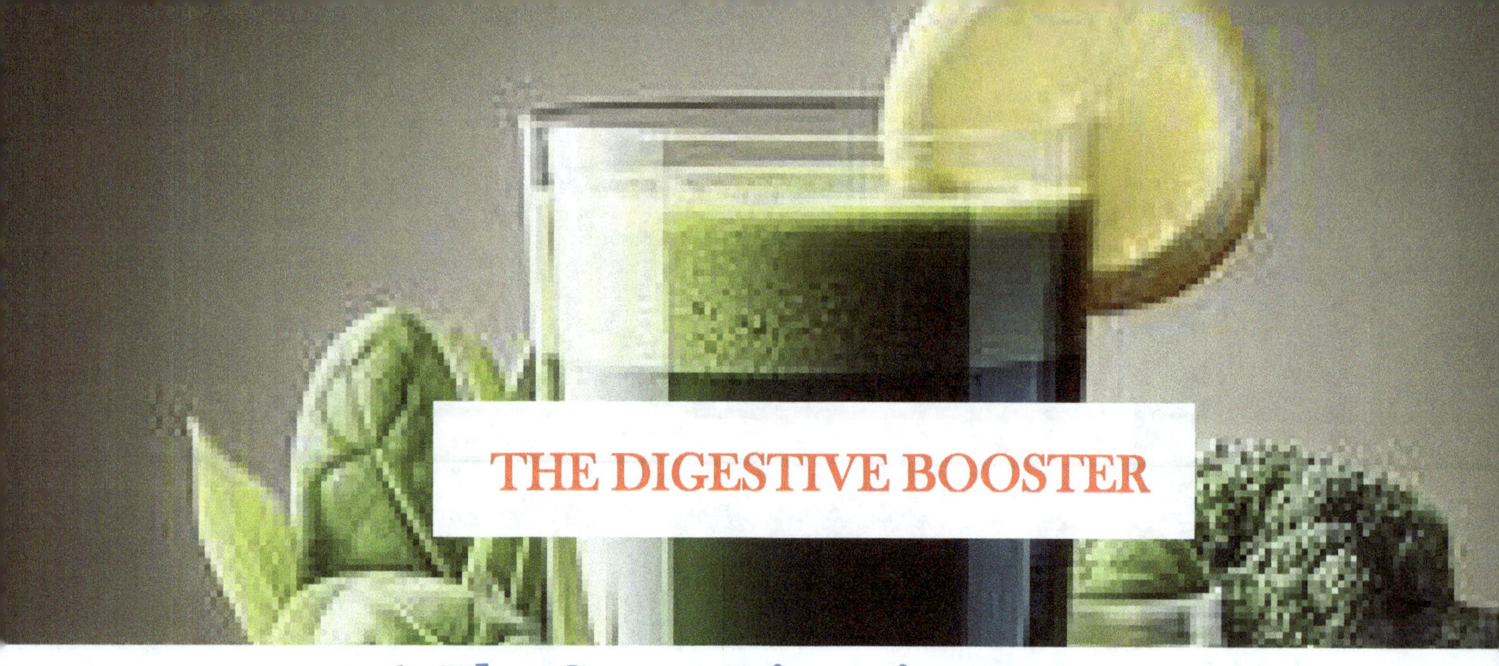

56. The Green Digestive Detox

Introduction:

This juice is packed with lush green veggies, which are high in nutrients such as vitamins, minerals, and antioxidants that can aid in cleansing the digestive system and improve digestion. The ginger and lemon in this juice also have digestive-boosting properties.

Ingredients:

1 cup kale

1 cup spinach

1/2 cucumber

1/2 peeled and chopped inch ginger root

1/4 lemon, peeled and juiced

Instructions:

Wash all of the ingredients well.

Cut the cucumber into small pieces.

Add all of the ingredients to a juicer and blend until smooth.

Serve immediately.

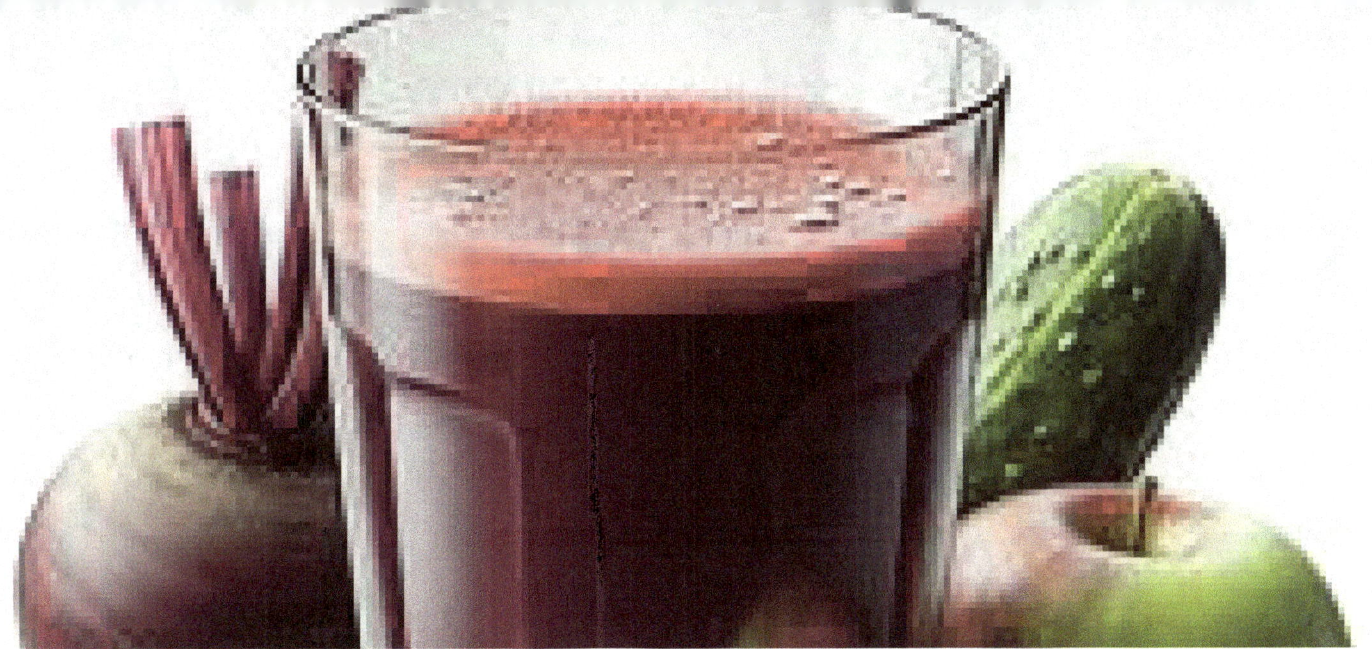

57. The Beet and Ginger Boost

Introduction:

This juice is packed with beets and ginger, both known for their digestive-boosting properties. Beets are a good source of fiber and potassium, which can help to regulate digestion. Ginger is known to help reduce inflammation and nausea.

Ingredients:

1 beet

1/2 inch peeled and chopped ginger root

1 apple

1/2 cucumber

1/2 cup water

Instructions:

Wash all of the ingredients well.

Cut the beet, apple, and cucumber into small pieces.

Add all of the ingredients to a juicer and blend until smooth.

Serve immediately.

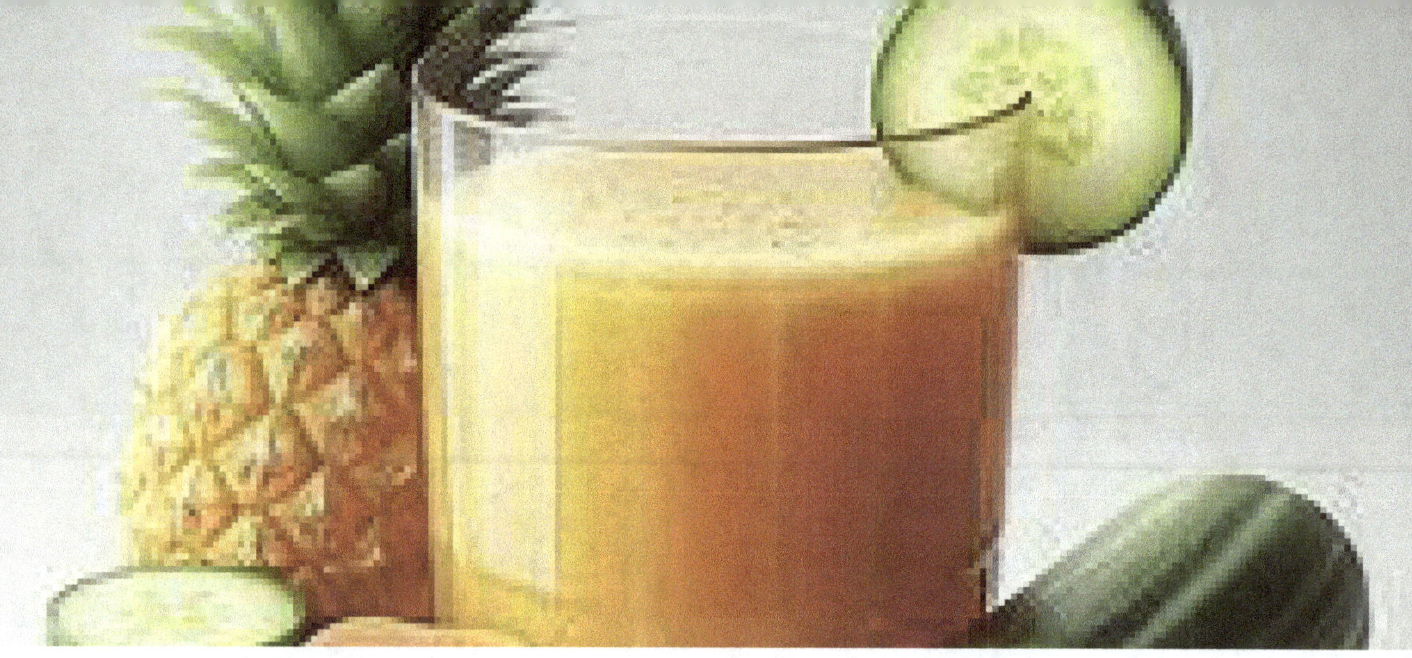

58. The Pineapple Papaya Cleanser

Introduction:

This juice is packed with pineapple and papaya, both known for their digestive-boosting enzymes. Bromelain, found in pineapple, aids in the breakdown of proteins, while papaya contains papain, which helps break down fats and carbohydrates.

Ingredients:

1 cup pineapple

1 cup papaya

1/2 cucumber

1/2 cup coconut water

Instructions:

Wash all of the ingredients well.

Cut the pineapple, papaya, and cucumber into small pieces.

Add all of the ingredients to a juicer and blend until smooth.

Serve immediately.

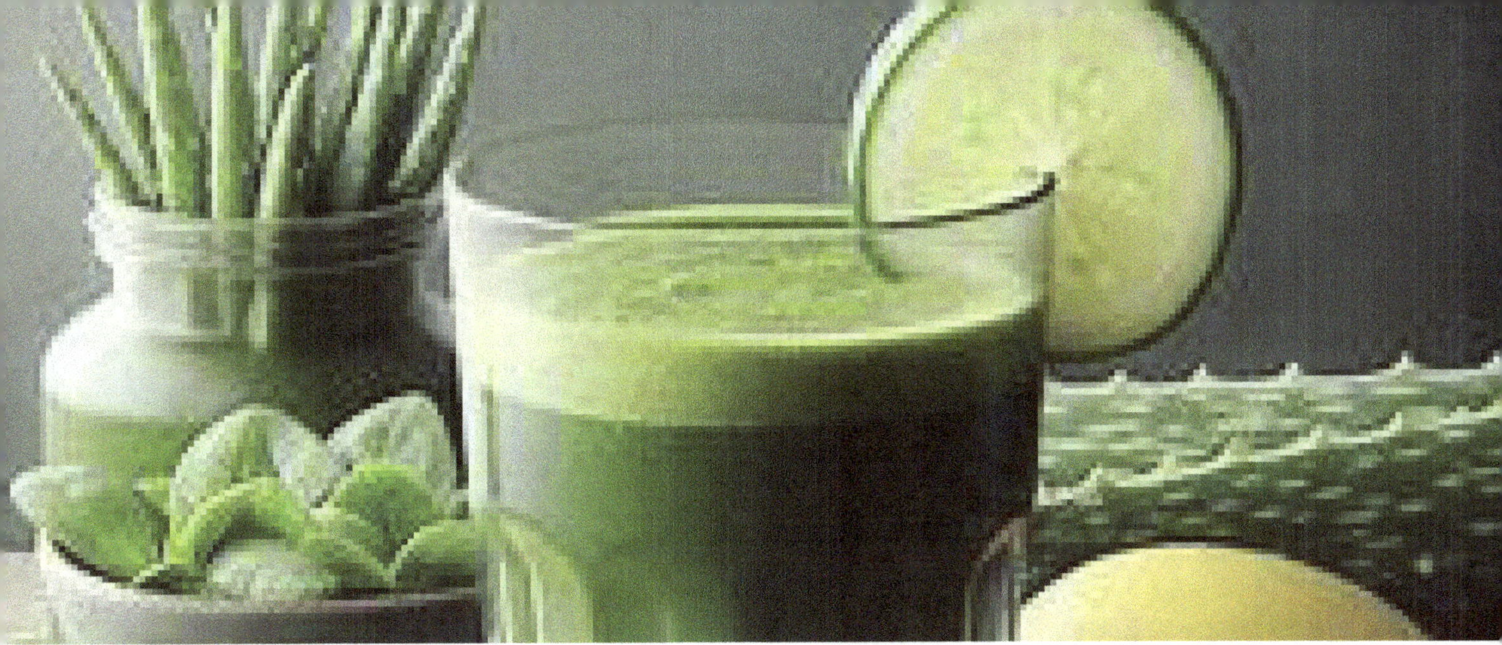

59. The Aloe Vera Digest Juice

Introduction:

This juice is packed with aloe vera, which has been shown to have digestive-boosting properties. Aloe vera is rich in fiber and prebiotics, which can assist in the promotion of healthy gut microorganisms.

Ingredients:

1/2 cup aloe vera juice

1 cup spinach

1/2 cucumber

1/2 lemon, peeled and juiced

Instructions:

In a blender, add all the ingredients and mix until smooth.

Serve immediately.

   Juicing for Cancer Recipes for Seniors

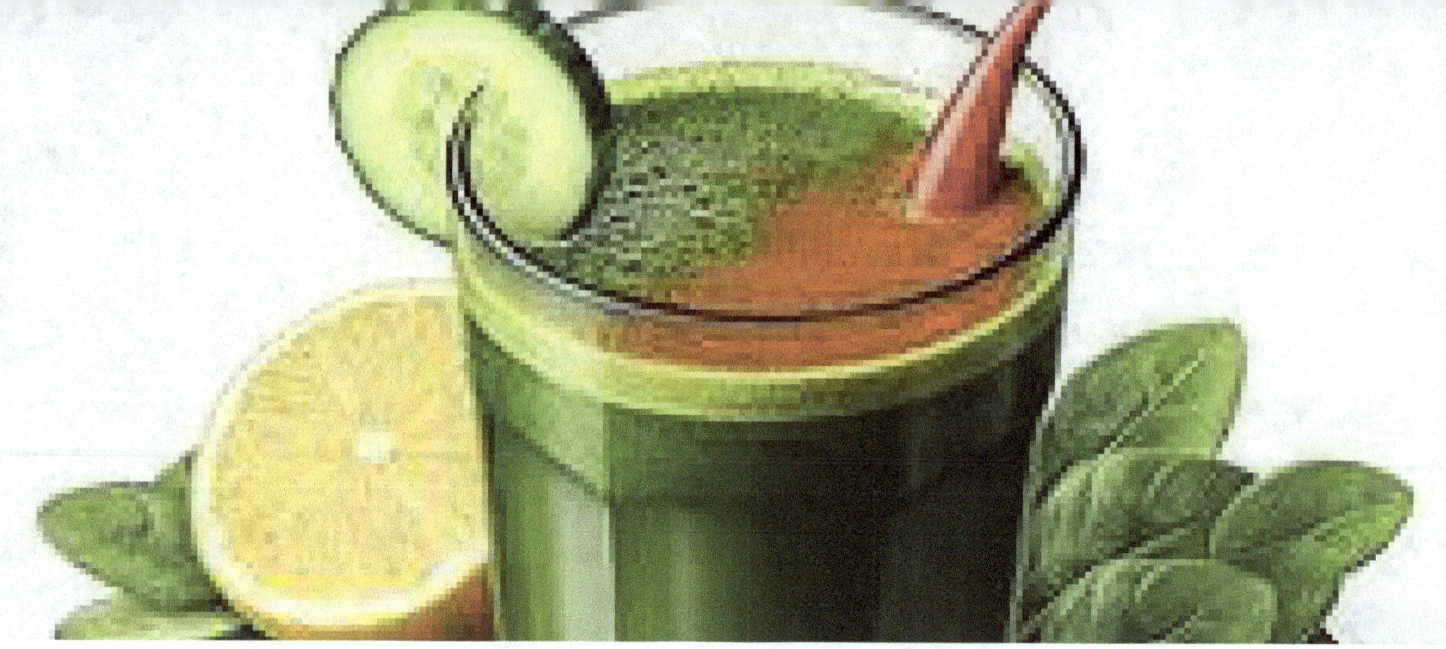

60. The Spicy Detox Juice

Introduction:

This juice is packed with cayenne pepper, which has been shown to have digestive-boosting properties. Cayenne pepper has been shown to increase the creation of digestive juices and blood flow to the digestive tract.

Ingredients:

1/4 teaspoon cayenne pepper

1 cup spinach

1/2 cucumber

1/2 lemon, peeled and juiced

1/2 cup water

Instructions:

In a blender, add all the

ingredients and mix until

smooth.

Serve immediately.

Juicing for Cancer Recipes for Seniors

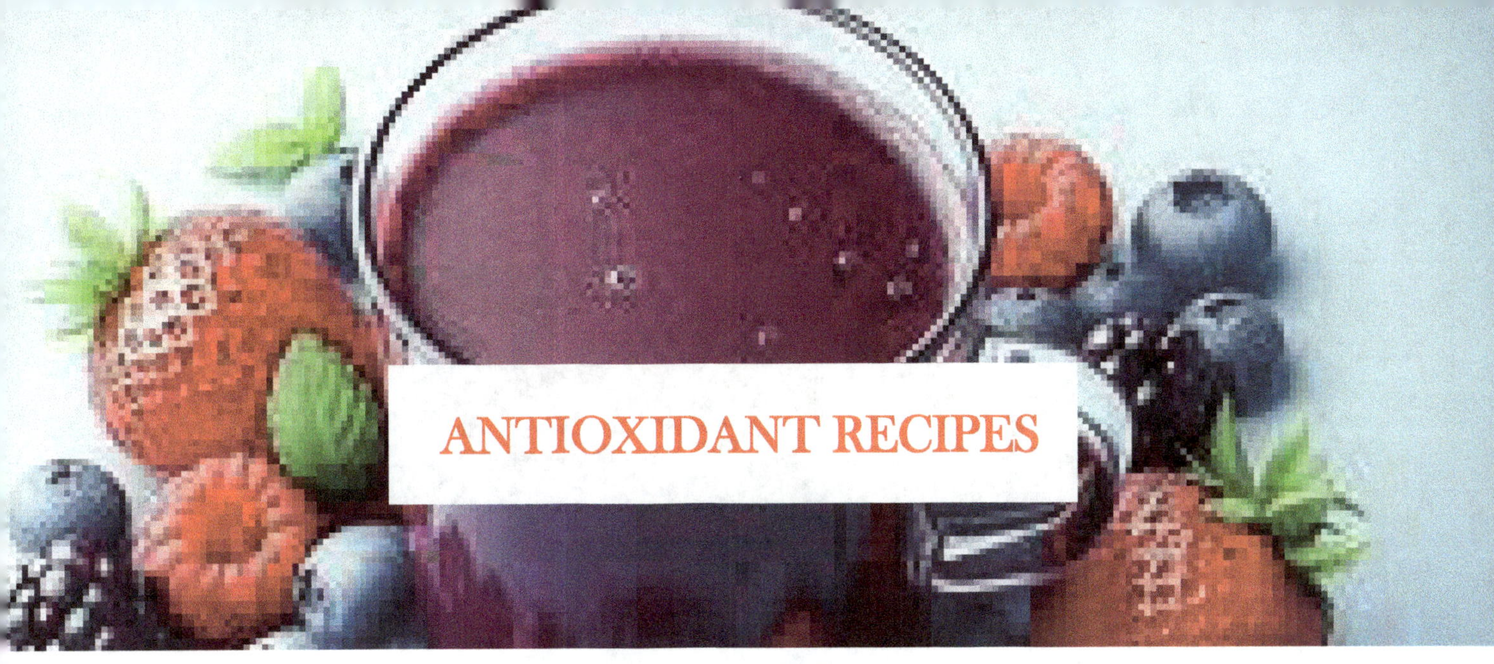

61. The Berry Blast

Introduction:

This juice is packed with berries, some of the most antioxidant-rich foods on the planet. Berries are rich in anthocyanins, powerful antioxidants that are capable of helping prevent cell damage.

Ingredients:

1 cup blueberries

1 cup strawberries

1/2 cup raspberries

1/2 cup blackberries

1/2 cup water

Instructions:

Wash all of the ingredients well.

Add all of the ingredients to a juicer and blend until smooth.

Serve immediately.

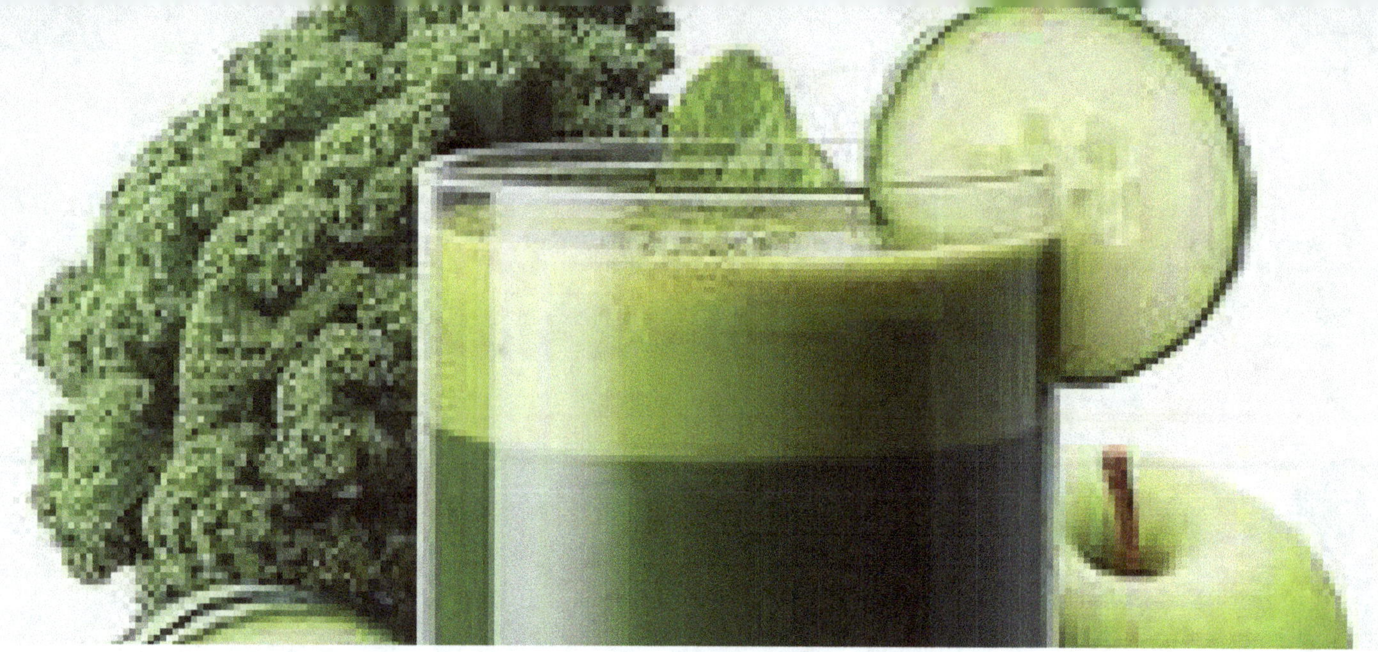

62. The Green Machine

Introduction:

This juice is packed with leafy green vegetables, a good source of antioxidants, vitamins, and minerals. Leafy green vegetables are high in carotenoids and antioxidants, which can help stop cancer and cardiovascular disease.

Ingredients:

1 cup kale

1 cup spinach

1/2 cucumber

1/2 green apple

1/2 cup water

Instructions:

Wash all of the ingredients well.

Cut the cucumber and apple

into small pieces.

Add all of the ingredients to a

juicer and blend until smooth.

Serve immediately

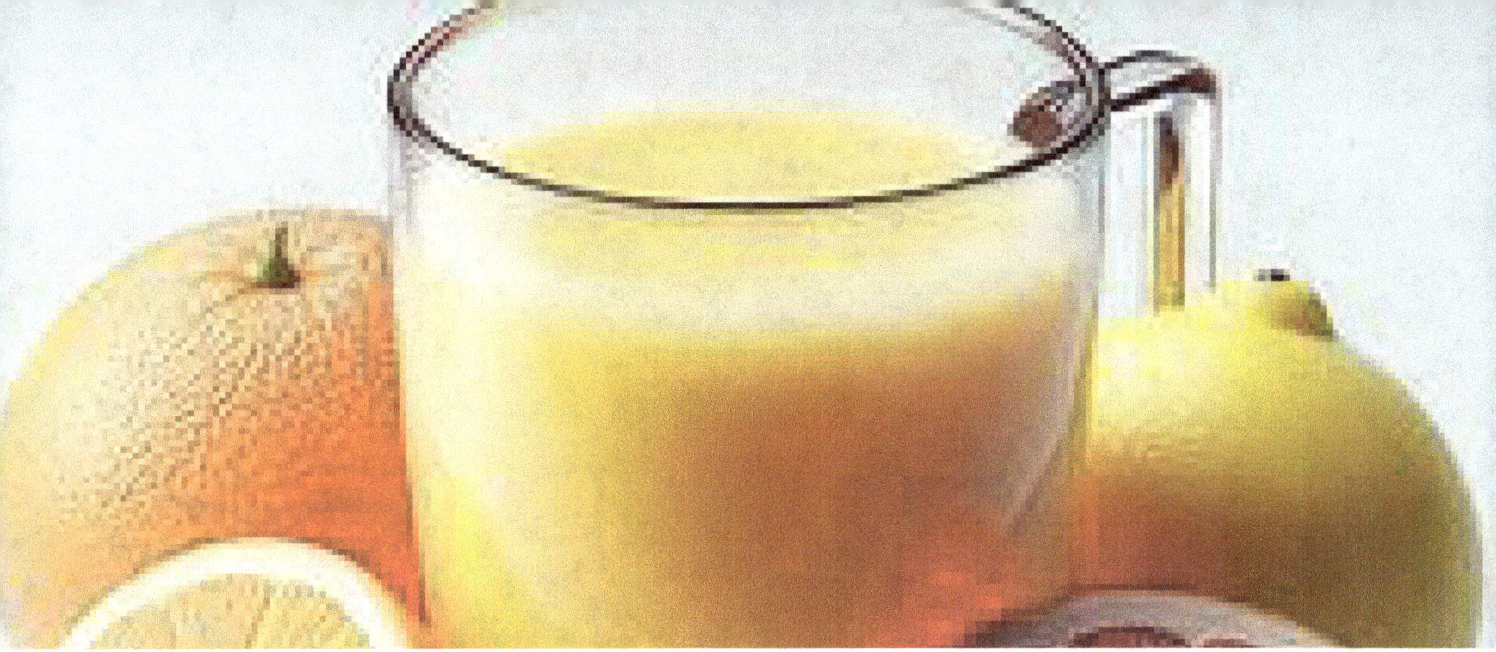

63. The Citrus Kick Juice

Introduction:

This juice is packed with fruits such as citrus, which are high in vitamin C and other antioxidants. Fruits rich in vitamin C contain a potent antioxidant that can protect the body against cell damage and boost the immune system.

Ingredients:

1 orange

1 grapefruit

1 lemon

1/2 cup water

Instructions:

Wash all of the ingredients well.

Cut the orange, grapefruit, and lemon into small pieces.

Add all of the ingredients to a juicer and blend until smooth.

Serve immediately.

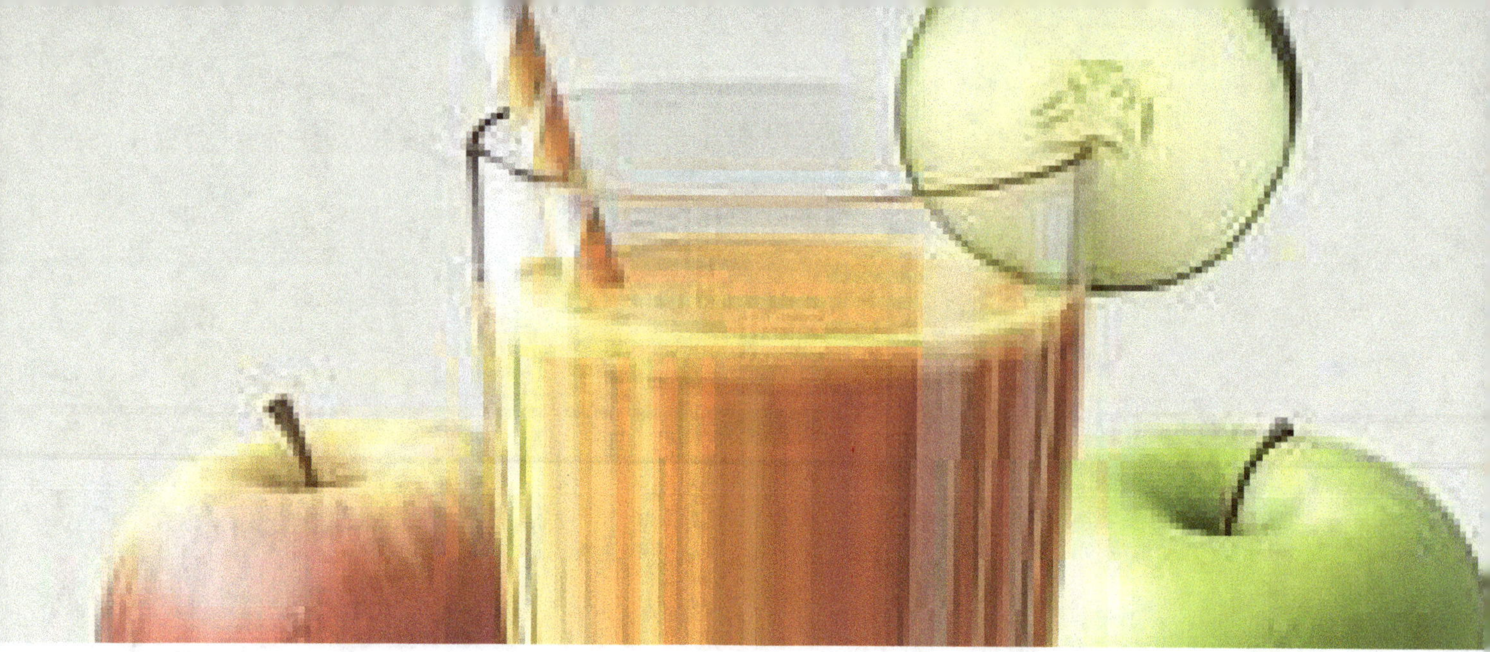

64. The Turmeric Boost Juice

Introduction:

This drink contains turmeric, a spice with potent anti-inflammatory and antioxidant qualities. Turmeric is known to help protect against cancer, heart disease, and Alzheimer's disease.

Ingredients:

1/2 inch turmeric root, peeled and chopped

1 carrot

1 apple

1/2 cucumber

1/2 cup water

Instructions:

Wash all of the ingredients well.

Cut the carrot, apple, and cucumber into small pieces.

Add all of the ingredients to a juicer and blend until smooth.

Serve immediately.

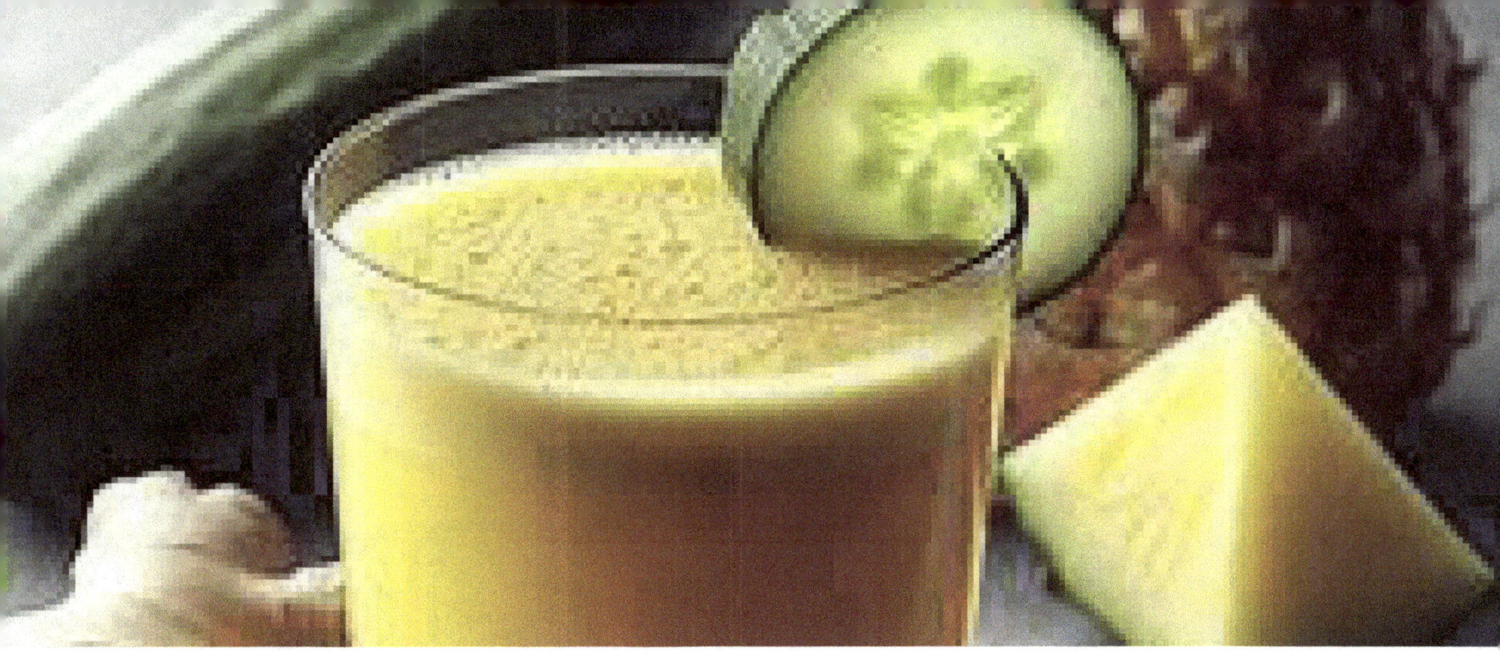

65. The Ginger Glow

Introduction:

This juice contains turmeric, a spice with potent anti-inflammatory and antioxidant qualities. Ginger is known to help reduce inflammation, boost the immune system, and improve digestion.

Ingredients:

1/2 inch peeled and chopped ginger root

1 pineapple

1/2 cucumber

1/2 cup coconut water

Instructions:

Wash all of the ingredients well.

Slice the pineapple and cucumber into tiny pieces.

Add all of the ingredients to a juicer and blend until smooth.

Serve immediately.

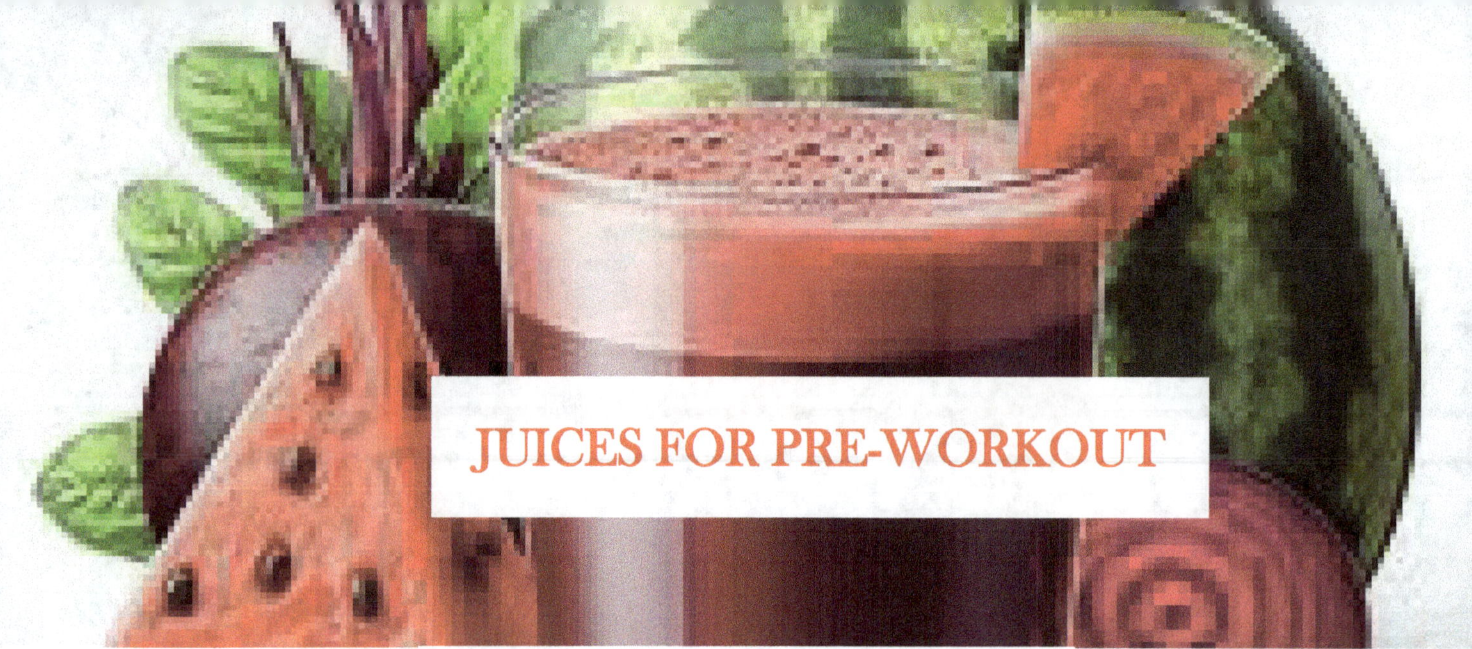

The Pump-Up Portion

Introduction:

This juice is packed with nitrates and antioxidants, which may be helpful in the enhancement of blood circulation and oxygen delivery to your muscles, boosting energy and endurance during your workout. Beetroot, watermelon, and ginger are good sources of minerals, such as potassium, vitamins and magnesium.

Ingredients:

1 beetroot, peeled and diced

2 cups watermelon, cubed

1-inch ginger root, peeled and chopped

Instructions:

Wash all of the ingredients well.

Cut the beetroot and watermelon into small pieces.

Add all of the ingredients to a juicer and blend until smooth.

Serve immediately.

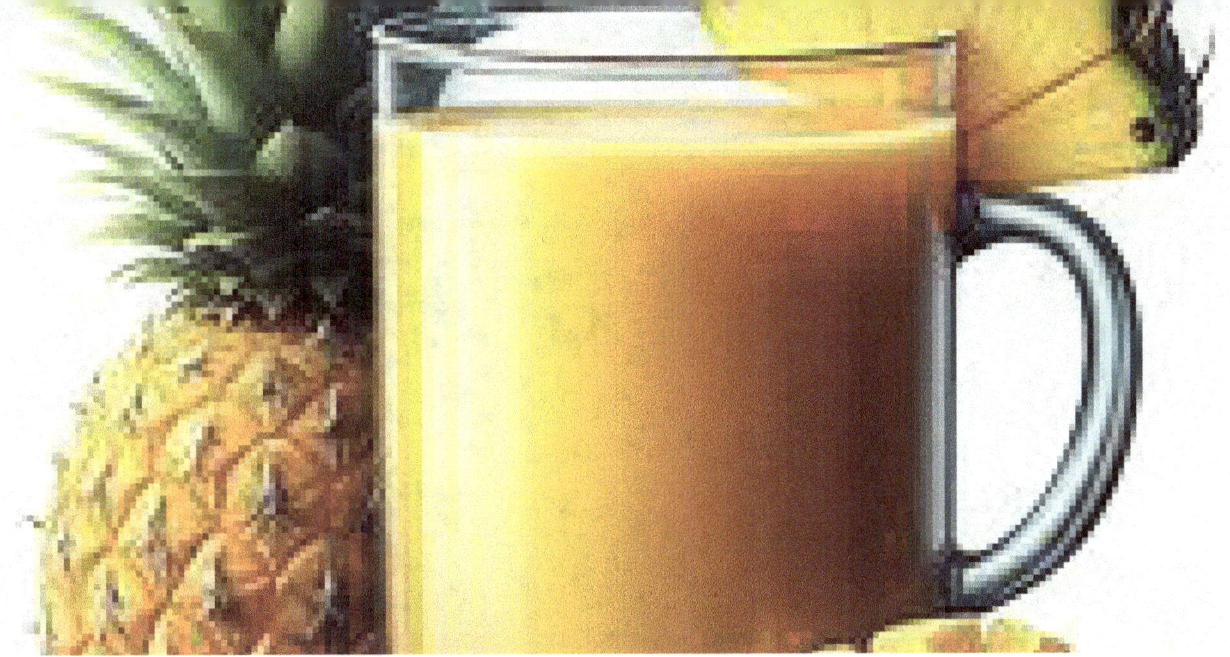

67. The Tropical Twist

Introduction:

This juice is a delicious and refreshing way to get your pre-workout boost. The pineapple and mango provide vitamins A and C and electrolytes. The coconut water adds electrolytes and MCTs, a type of fat that can be used for energy. The turmeric and black pepper add anti-inflammatory and antioxidant properties.

Ingredients:

1 cup pineapple, diced

1 cup mango, diced

1 cup coconut water

1/4 inch turmeric root, peeled and chopped

1/4 teaspoon black pepper

Instructions:

Wash all of the ingredients well.

Cut the pineapple and mango into small pieces.

Add all of the ingredients to a juicer and blend until smooth.

Serve immediately.

   Juicing for Cancer Recipes for Seniors

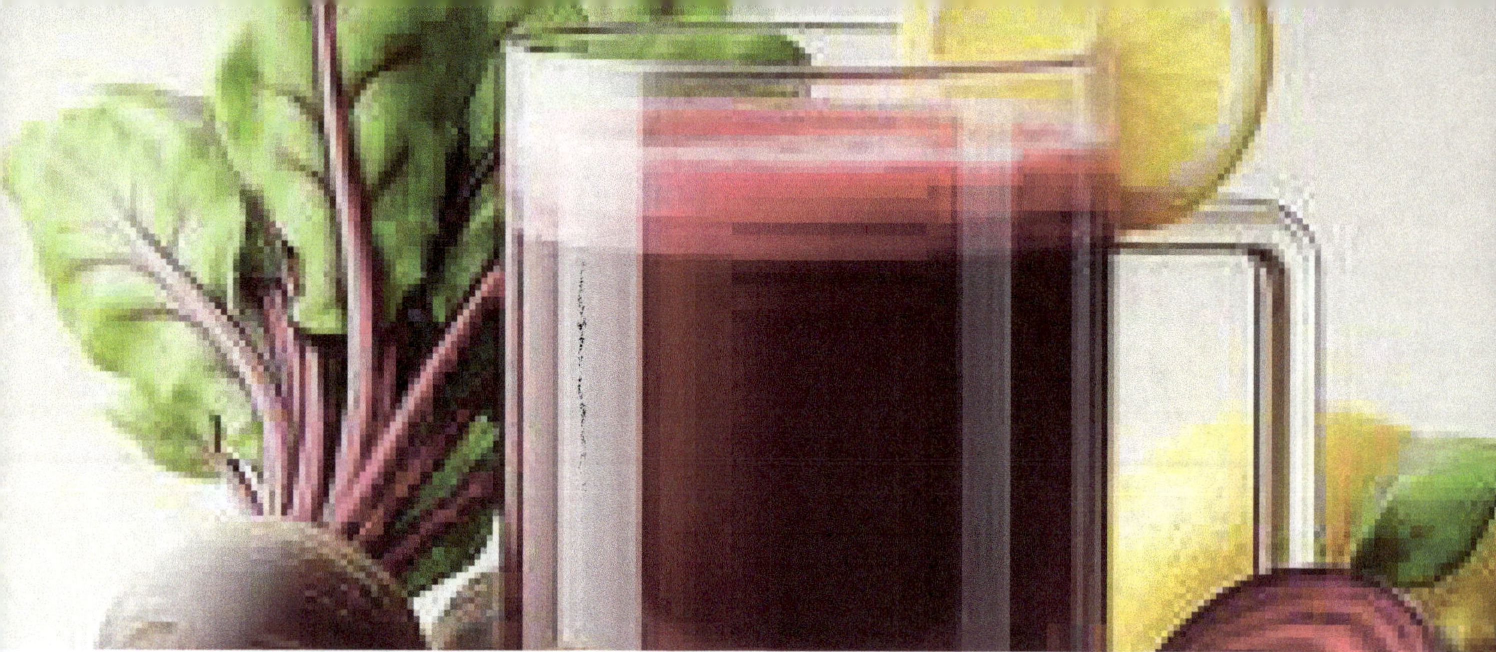

68. The Beetroot Booster

Introduction:

This juice is packed with beetroot, a good source of nitrates and antioxidants. Nitrates can help enhance blood flow and oxygen supply to your muscle tissue, providing energy and endurance during your workout. The ginger and lemon add a kick of flavor and heat.

Ingredients:

2 beets, peeled and diced

1-inch ginger root, peeled and chopped

1/2 lemon, juiced

Instructions:

Wash all of the ingredients well.

Cut the beets and ginger into small pieces.

Add all of the ingredients to a juicer and blend until smooth.

Serve immediately.

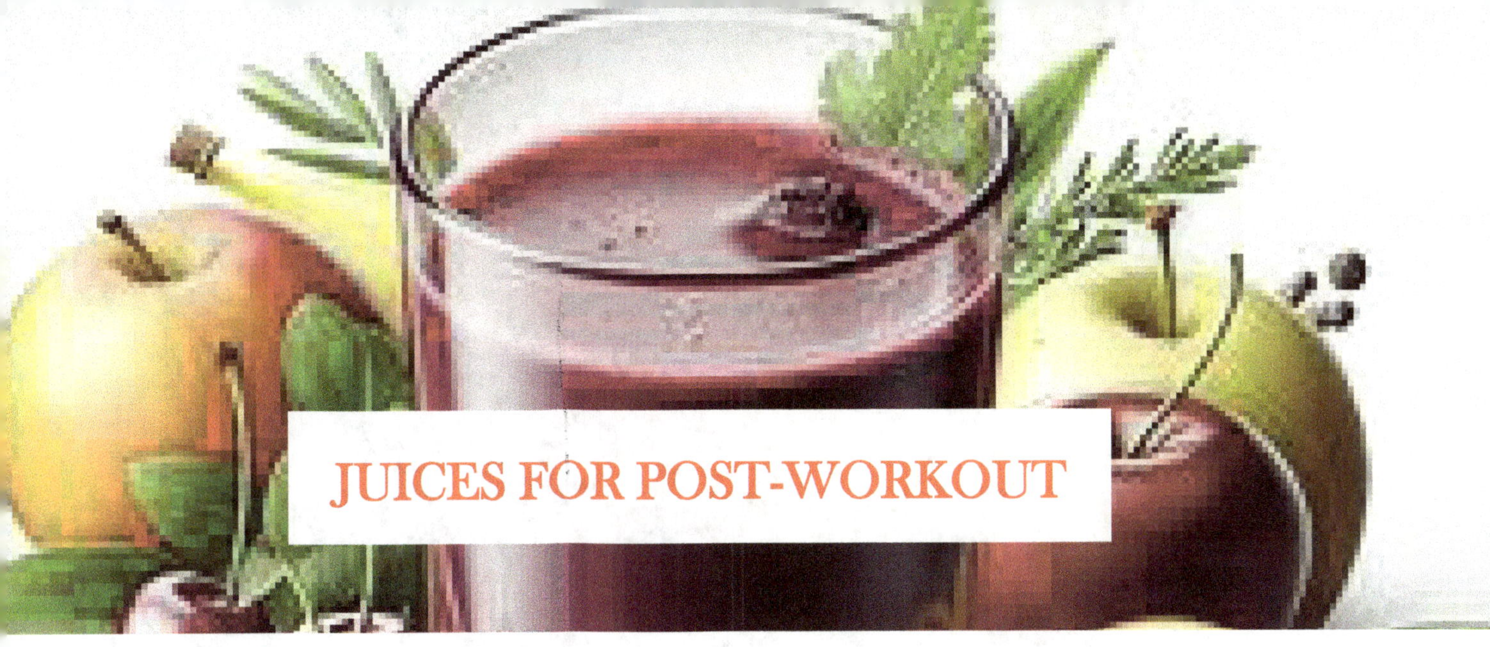

69. The Muscle Mender Juice

Introduction:

This juice contains nutrients and electrolytes to help your muscles recover after a challenging workout. The tart cherry juice is a good source of antioxidants and anti-inflammatory compounds. At the same time, coconut water provides electrolytes and MCTs, a type of fat that can be used for energy. And the turmeric and black pepper add anti-inflammatory and antioxidant properties.

Ingredients:

1 cup tart cherry juice

1 cup coconut water

1/4 inch turmeric root, peeled and chopped

1/4 teaspoon black pepper

Instructions:

Wash all of the ingredients well.

Add all of the ingredients to a juicer and blend until smooth.

Serve immediately.

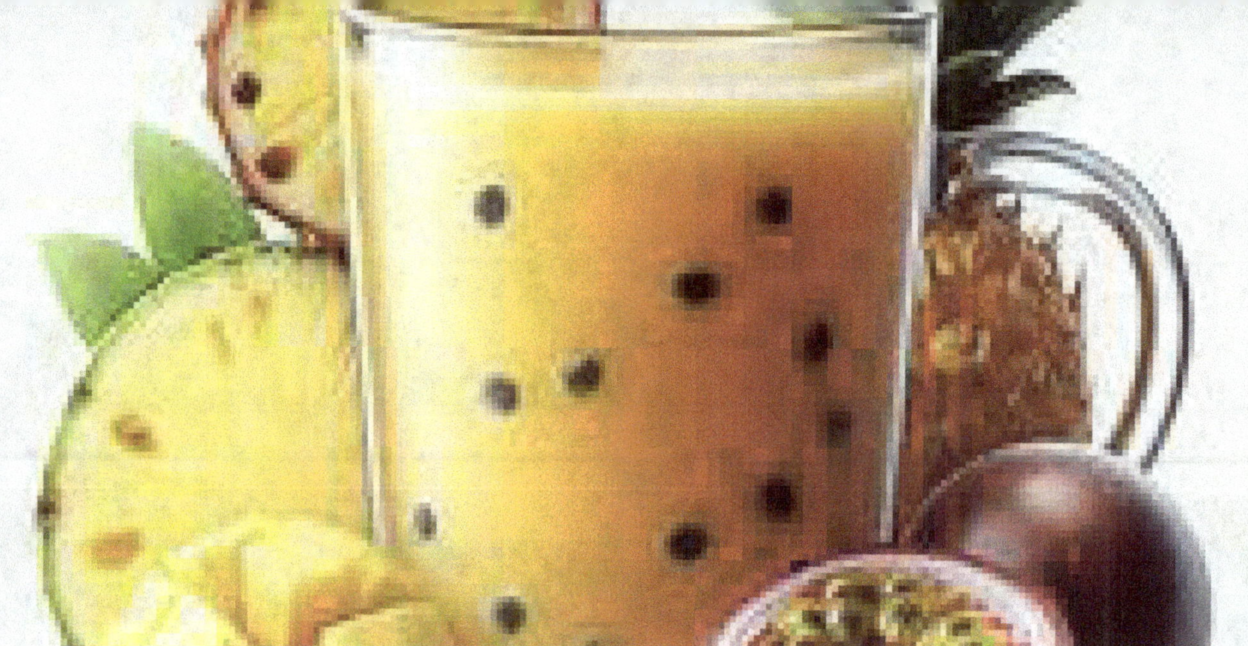

70. The Tropical Recovery

Introduction:

This juice is a delicious and refreshing way to refuel your body after a workout. The pineapple and mango provide vitamins A and C and electrolytes. The coconut water adds electrolytes and MCTs, a type of fat that can be used for energy. The passion fruit and guava add a sweet and exotic

Ingredients:

1 cup pineapple, diced

1 cup mango, diced

1 cup coconut water

1 passion fruit, halved and scooped

1/2 guava, peeled and seeded

Instructions:

Wash all of the ingredients well.

Cut the pineapple, mango, passion fruit, and guava into small pieces.

Add all of the ingredients to a juicer and blend until smooth.

Serve immediately.

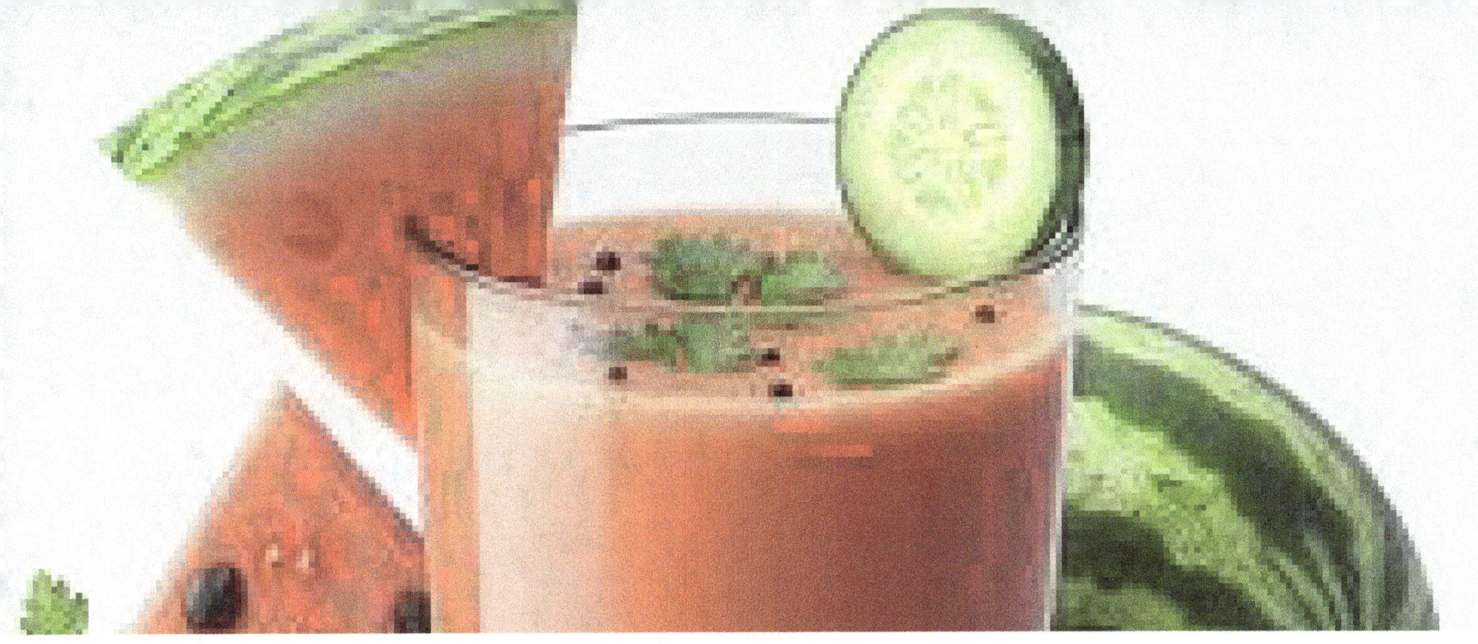

71. The Watermelon Warrior

Introduction:

This juice is packed with watermelon, a good source of electrolytes and antioxidants. Watermelon is also a natural source of L-citrulline, which can assist in enhancing the circulation of blood and lessen muscular weakness. The cucumber and ginger add hydration and flavor.

Ingredients:

2 cups watermelon, cubed

1 cucumber, peeled and diced

1-inch ginger root, peeled and chopped

Instructions:

Wash all of the ingredients well.

Cut the watermelon and cucumber into small pieces.

Add all of the ingredients to a juicer and blend until smooth.

Serve immediately.

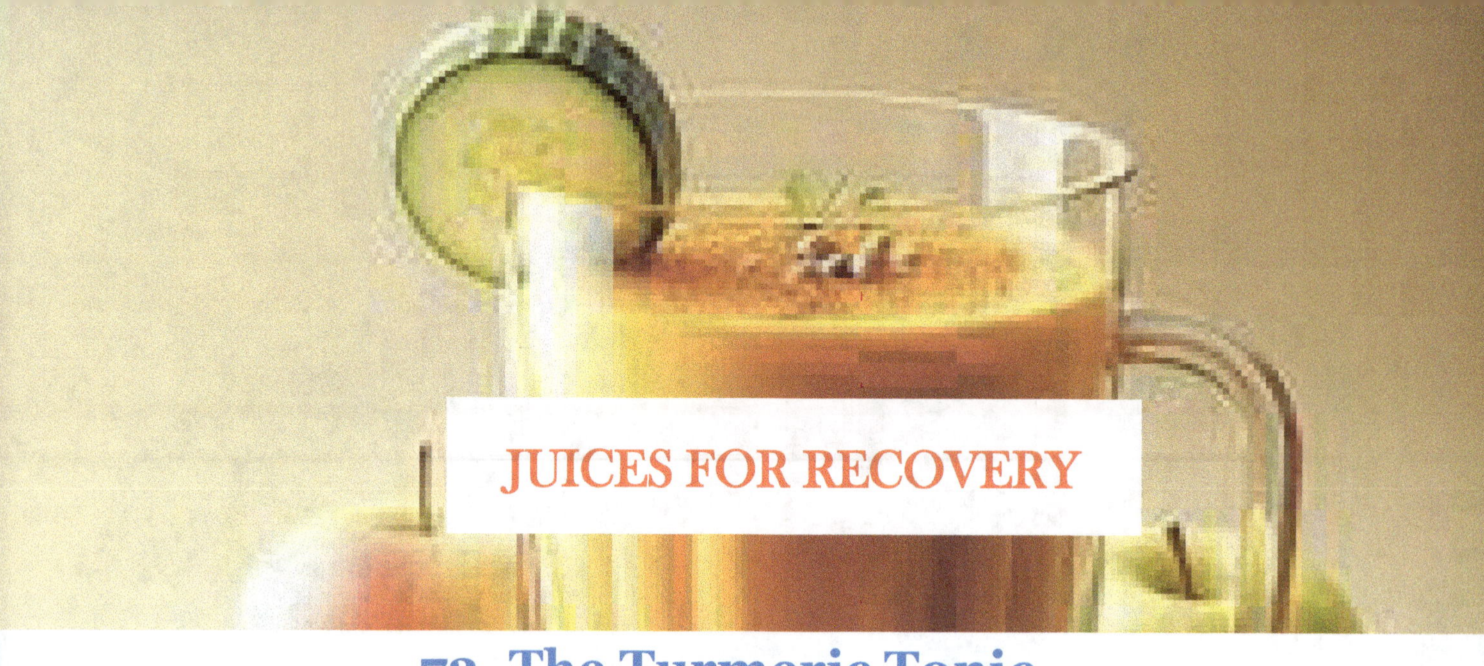

72. The Turmeric Tonic

Introduction:

This juice contains turmeric, a potent anti-inflammatory and antioxidant. Turmeric can help to reduce inflammation, improve muscle recovery, and boost the immune system. The ginger and black pepper enhance the absorption of the turmeric's curcumin. The orange and pineapple add sweetness and flavor.

Ingredients:

1/2 inch turmeric root, peeled and chopped

1/2 inch peeled and chopped ginger root

1/4 teaspoon black pepper

1 orange, peeled and segmented

1 cup pineapple, diced

Instructions:

Wash all of the ingredients well.

Cut the orange and pineapple into small pieces.

Add all of the ingredients to a juicer and blend until smooth.

Serve immediately.

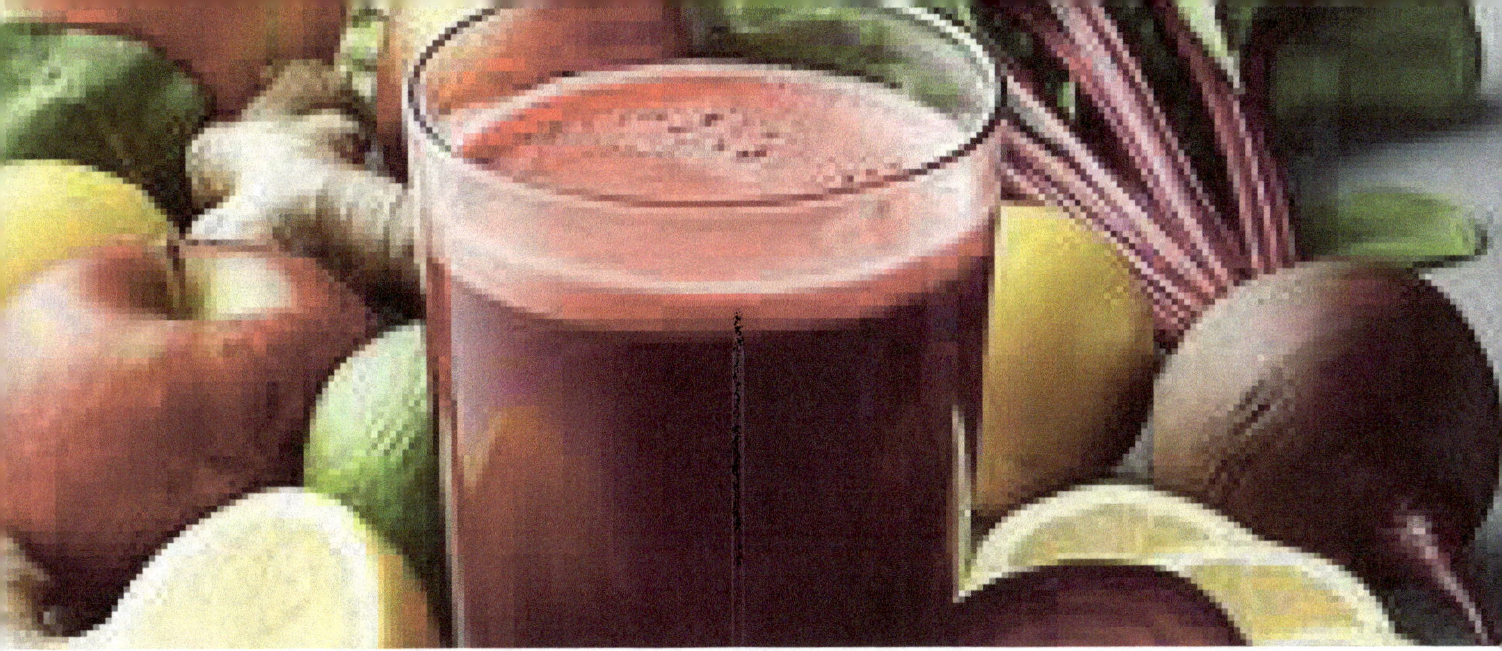

73. The Beet Blast Juice

Introduction:

Beets are a good source of nitrates, which can improve blood circulation and oxygen supply to the muscles, helping in recovery. The ginger and lemon add flavor and boost the absorption of nutrients.

Ingredients:

2 beets, peeled and diced

1-inch ginger root, peeled and chopped

1/2 lemon, juiced

Instructions:

Wash all of the ingredients well.

Cut the beets and ginger into small pieces.

Add all of the ingredients to a juicer and blend until smooth.

Serve immediately.

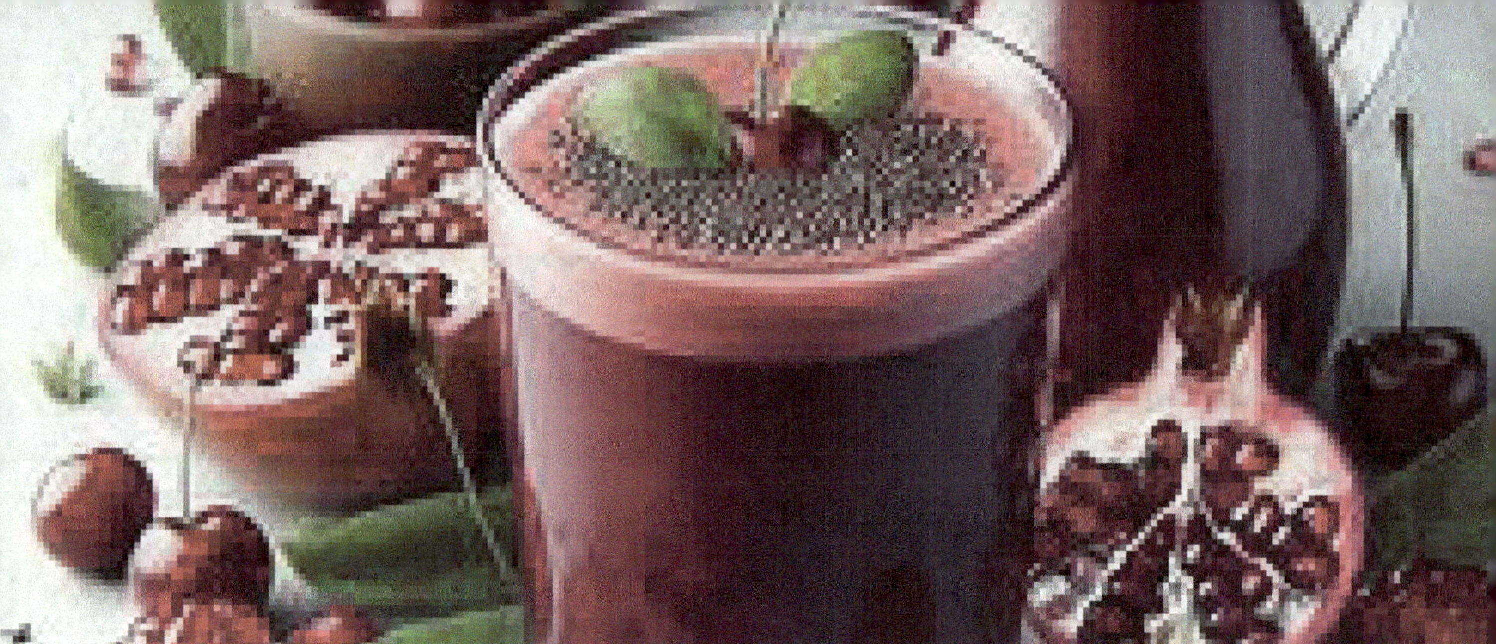

74. The Tart Cherry Tango Juice

Introduction:

Tart cherries are an excellent supply of anti-inflammatory and antioxidant qualities that can assist in reducing muscle soreness and improve recovery. The pomegranate and chia seeds add sweetness, fiber, and omega-3 fatty acids.

Ingredients:

1 cup tart cherry juice

1/2 cup pomegranate juice

1 tablespoon chia seeds

1/2 cup water

Instructions:

Wash all of the ingredients well.

Include the ingredients in a blender and blend until smooth.

Serve immediately.

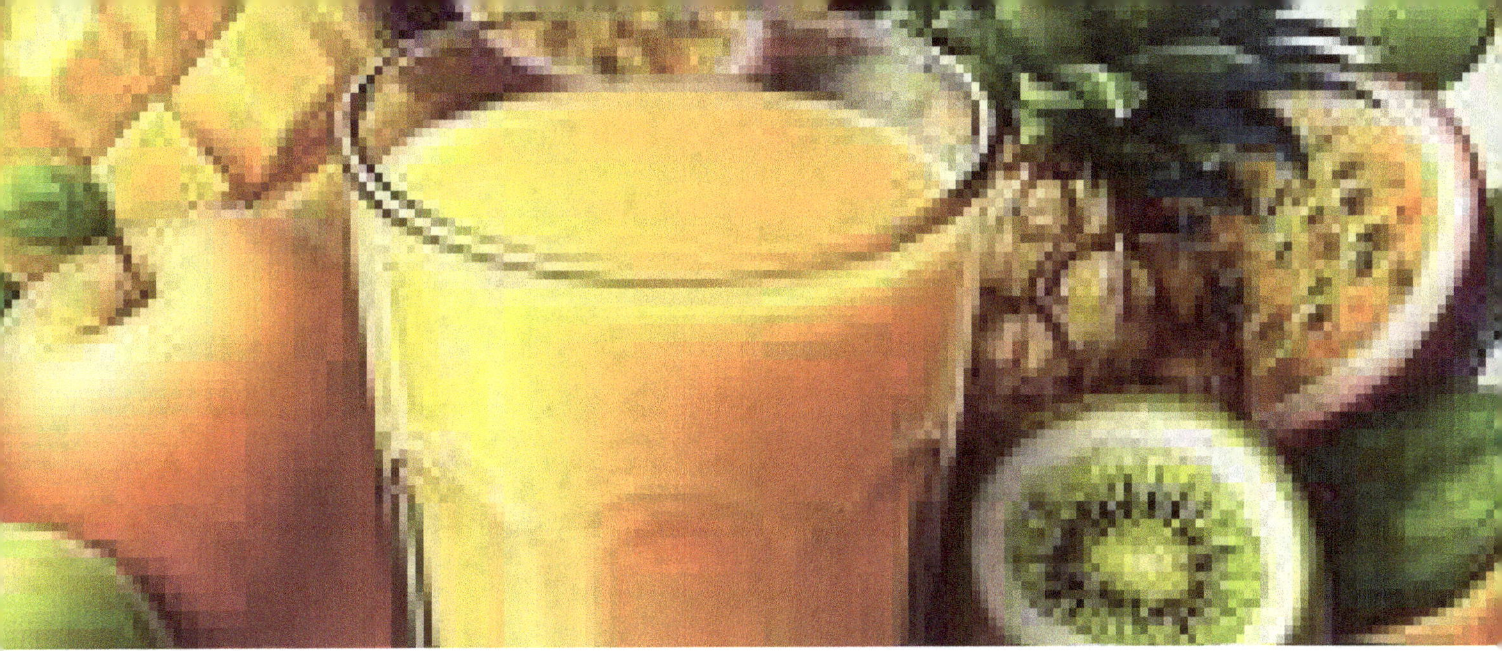

75. The Tropical Oasis

Introduction:

This juice is packed with tropical fruits, a good source of vitamins, minerals, and antioxidants. The pineapple, mango, and coconut water also provide electrolytes and MCTs, a type of fat that can be used for energy. This juice can help to replenish your body's nutrients and electrolytes after a challenging workout, and it's also a delicious and refreshing way to cool down.

Ingredients:

1 cup pineapple, diced

1 cup mango, diced

1 cup coconut water

1 passion fruit, halved and scooped

1/2 guava, peeled and seeded

Instructions:

Wash all of the ingredients well.

Cut the pineapple, mango, passion fruit, and guava into small pieces.

Add all of the ingredients to a juicer and blend until smooth.

Serve immediately.

   Juicing for Cancer Recipes for Seniors

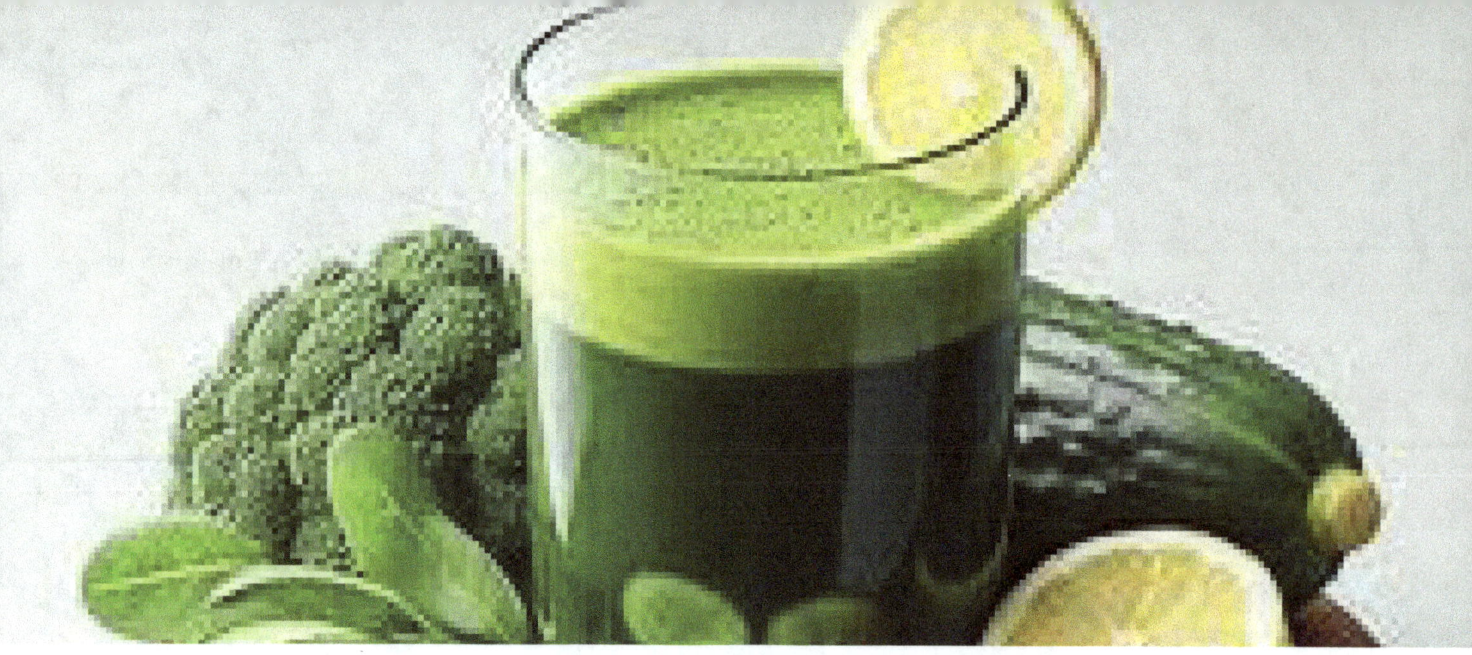

76. Green Goddess Juice

Introduction:

This juice is packed with leafy greens and other vegetables, a good source of vitamins, minerals, and antioxidants. The spinach, kale, and celery also provide electrolytes. The cucumber and ginger add hydration and flavour. This juice can help to replenish your body's nutrients and electrolytes after a challenging workout, and it's also an excellent way to get your daily dose of greens.

Ingredients:

1 cup spinach

1 cup kale

1/2 cup celery, chopped

1 cucumber, peeled and diced

1-inch ginger root, peeled and chopped

Instructions:

Wash all of the ingredients well.

Cut the cucumber and ginger into small pieces.

Add all of the ingredients to a juicer and blend until smooth.

Serve immediately.

CONCLUSION

Congratulations, you have completed this book, and I hope you have gained a lot of valuable insights about the benefits of juicing for seniors, especially those facing cancer or undergoing cancer treatment. Juicing can help cleanse your body and remove toxins by providing antioxidants, chlorophyll, and sulfur compounds that can fight off free radicals, eliminate heavy metals, and boost liver function.

Juicing can also help hydrate and nourish your body, strengthen your immune system, ward off infections, lower your blood pressure, enhance blood circulation, reduce inflammation, and prevent cell damage. Juicing can also help improve your digestion, skin, hair, and mood, which may be affected by the adverse effects of radiation or chemotherapy treatment.

I have shared several juice recipes in this book to help cleanse your body and support your immune system. These juices are high in antioxidant substances, minerals, vitamins, and other nu and phytochemicals that can guard against oxidative stress, inflammatory disorders, and DNA damage. They are also easy to prepare and tasty to drink. You can use a juicer or a blender to make these juices, but wash the fruits and vegetables well before juicing. You can also modify the amount of ingredients according to your liking and preference.

Try the recipes in this book and experiment with your combinations of fruits and vegetables. You can create juice recipes based on your favorite flavors, colors, and health goals. You can also add other ingredients such as herbs, spices, nuts, seeds, or supplements to improve the taste and nutrition of your juices. The possibilities are endless!

However, before you embark on any juicing regimen, please consult your doctor or dietitian first. Juicing may not be appropriate for everyone, especially if you have certain medical conditions or allergies. Juicing may also affect your blood sugar levels, blood pressure, and weight, so you need to monitor them regularly. Juicing should not replace your regular meals or medications but supplement them with a balanced diet.

 Juicing for Cancer Recipes for Seniors

Thank you for your interest in and support of this book. Like I loved writing it, I hope you enjoyed reading it too. I wish you good health and happiness in your juicing journey for cancer prevention and treatment. Remember, you are not alone in this battle. You have the power of nature on your side! Cheers!

Please share this book with your friends and family and leave an honest review if you enjoyed it. Your feedback and support are greatly appreciated!

Happy Juicing

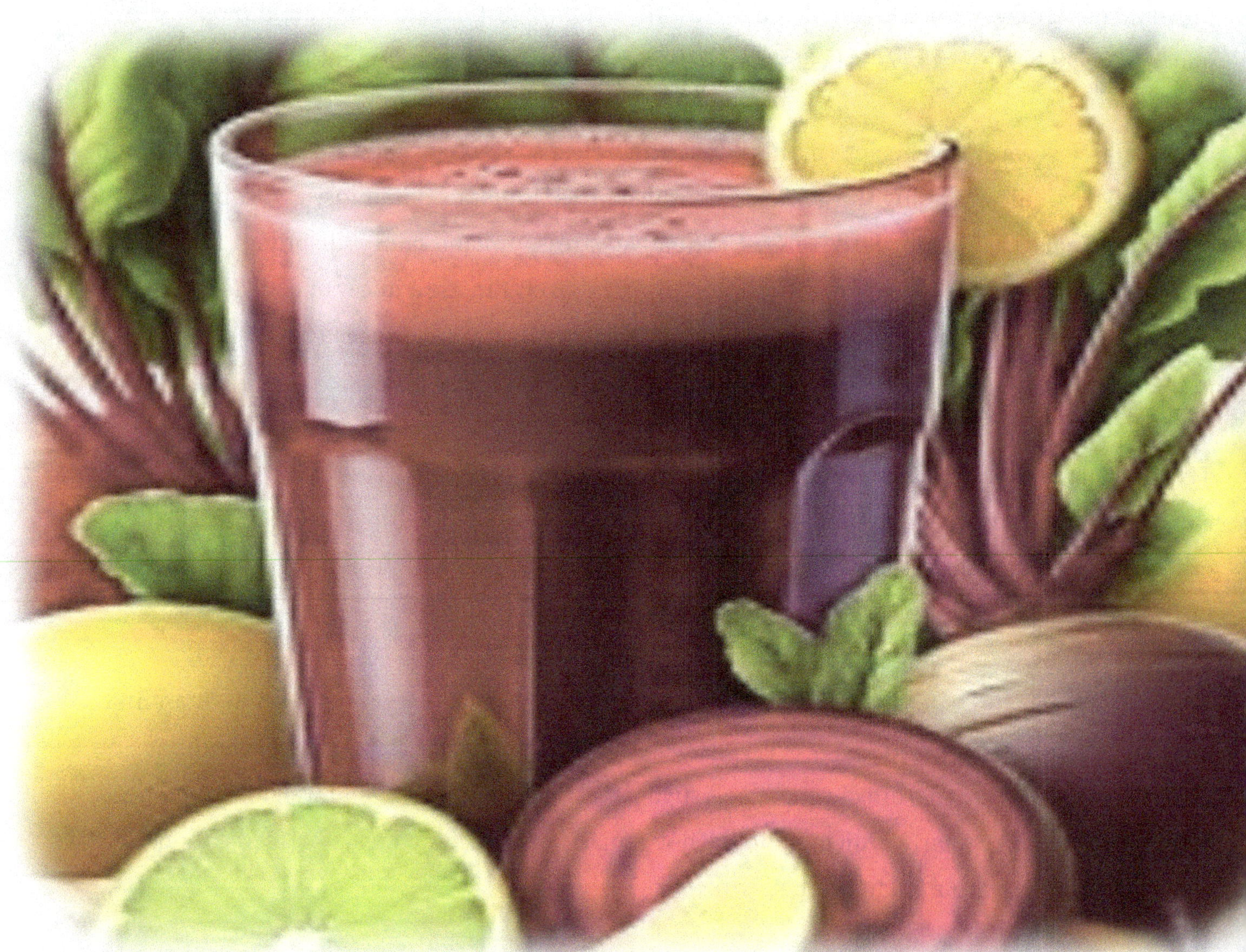

   Juicing for Cancer Recipes for Seniors